Aggression and Destructiver

T0264786

Aggression is a part of human nature that energises our relationships, acts as an impetus for psychic development, and enables us to master our world. More often, we focus on its more destructive aspects, such as the violence individuals inflict on themselves or others and overlook the positive functions of aggression.

In *Aggression and Destructiveness*, Celia Harding brings together contributions from experienced psychoanalysts and psychoanalytic psychotherapists to explore the roots of aggression and the clinical dilemmas it presents in psychotherapy. Beginning with accounts of aggression and destructiveness from a range of developmental and theoretical perspectives, the book provides useful insights into subjects including:

- Bullying and abusive relationships
- Male and female violence and destructiveness
- Depressive, perverse and psychotic states of mind
- Attacks on therapeutic treatment

This book makes a valuable contribution to the attempt to make sense of human aggression, destructiveness and violence perpetrated against the self, others and reality. It will be of great interest to trainee and qualified psychodynamic counsellors, psychoanalytic psychotherapists and psychoanalysts.

Celia Harding is a psychoanalytic psychotherapist in private practice in East London and editor of *Sexuality: Psychoanalytic Perspectives*.

Contributors: Anne Amos, Rose Christie, Celia Harding, Anne Harrison, Leon Kleimberg, Richard Lucas, David Mann, Marianne Parsons, Paul Renn, Robert Royston, Stanley Ruszczynski, Mary Thomas, John Woods

Aggression and Destructiveness

Psychoanalytic Perspectives

Edited by Celia Harding

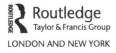

Routledge
Taylor & Francis Group

LONDON AND NEW YORK

Published 2006 by Routledge
27 Church Road, Hove, East Sussex BN3 2FA

Simultaneously published in the USA and Canada
by Routledge
711 Third Avenue, New York, NY 10017

Routledge is an imprint of the Taylor & Francis Group, an informa business

Typeset in Times by Garfield Morgan, Mumbles, Swansea

Paperback cover design by Lisa Dynan based on an idea by Andrew Harvey

British Library Cataloguing in Publication Data
A catalogue record for this book is available from the British Library

Library of Congress Cataloging in Publication Data
Aggression and destructiveness : psychoanalytic perspectives / edited by Celia Harding.
    p. cm.
   Includes bibliographical references and index.
   ISBN 1-58391-884-1 (alk. paper) – ISBN 1-58391-885-X (pbk. : alk. paper)
     1. Aggressiveness. 2. Self-destructive behavior. 3. Violence–Psychological
   aspects. I. Harding, Celia, 1955–

   RC569.5.A34A355 2006
   16.85'82–dc26
                                                                    2005043531

ISBN13: 978-1-58391-884-5 hbk
ISBN13: 978-1-58391-885-2 pbk

Contents

Contributors

Anne Amos is a member of the British Psycho-Analytical Society and currently works as a psychoanalyst in private practice in London as well as teaching and supervising within the heath service. Her original training was as a social worker and more recently she worked at the Tavistock Marital Studies Institute.

Rose Christie is a psychoanalytic psychotherapist member of the Foundation for Psychotherapy and Counselling. She is project manager of the 'Insight into Violence' project at the Maya Centre, based in North London, which offers free psychoanalytic therapy to local deprived women. The violence project seeks to address the need for treatment for women who have experienced significant levels of violence in their history, the majority of whom are in violent relationships at the time of referral.

Celia Harding is a psychoanalytic psychotherapist in private practice in East London. She trained with the Westminster Pastoral Foundation and she is a member and training therapist of the Foundation for Psychotherapy and Counselling. She organised post-qualification courses for FPC for 10 years. She is Convenor of the FPC Ethics Committee. She is a founder member of the Association for Psychotherapy in East London. She edited a selection of papers entitled *Sexuality: Psychoanalytic Perspectives* (Brunner-Routledge 2000).

Anne Harrison is a member of the British Psycho-Analytical Society and a child analyst. She works in private practice and is a member of the Directorate of the London Clinic of Psychoanalysis. Her background is in classics and intellectual history. She has been a member of staff at the Portman Clinic and has worked in community mental health. She teaches on several psychotherapy trainings, including the British Psycho-Analytical Society, and is an Honorary Senior Lecturer on the MSc course in Psychoanalytic Studies at University College London.

Leon Kleimberg is a training analyst for the British Psycho-Analytical Society and the British Association of Psychotherapists. He is in full-time private practice in London. He has published papers in UK journals and abroad. One of his main areas of interest is creativity and psychopathology.

Richard Lucas is Consultant Psychiatrist at St Ann's Hospital, London. He is a Fellow of the Royal College of Psychiatrists and a Member of the British Psycho-Analytical Society. He is chair of the general psychiatry section of the Association for Psychoanalytic Psychotherapy in the NHS. He has written and lectured widely on topics related to psychosis, including the psychotic wavelength, cyclical psychoses, puerperal psychosis, risk assessment and psychosis workshops. He received the OBE in 2003 for psychiatric service to the Disability Living Allowance Advisory Board.

David Mann is a psychoanalytic psychotherapist and a member of the London Centre for Psychotherapy. He is Principal Psychotherapist at the NHS Psychotherapy Service based in Tunbridge Wells, Kent. He is also in private practice as a psychotherapist and supervisor in Tunbridge Wells and South London. He previously trained as an art therapist and worked in a variety of psychiatric and therapeutic communities. He lectures, teaches and runs workshops around the UK and Europe and has published extensively in leading national and international journals. He is author of *Psychotherapy: An Erotic Relationship – Transference and Countertransference Passions* (Routledge 1997) which was also translated and published in Germany in 1999 by the Klett-Cotta Press and he is the editor of *Erotic Transference and Countertransference: Clinical Practice in Psychotherapy* (Routledge 1999) and *Love and Hate: Psychoanalytic Perspectives* (Brunner-Routledge 2002).

Marianne Parsons is a psychoanalyst, a child analyst and a child psychotherapist. She trained at the Anna Freud Centre and the British Psycho-Analytical Society. She was Head of the Clinical Training at the Anna Freud Centre and Joint Editor of the *Journal of Child Psychotherapy*. She has a private practice and also works in the NHS at the Portman Clinic in London. She is visiting lecturer in child and adolescent development and psychoanalytic technique in Oula, Finland, and in Tampa, Florida.

Paul Renn is a psychoanalytic psychotherapist in private practice in West London. He is a member of the Centre for Attachment-based Psychoanalytic Psychotherapy (CAPP), where he is on the teaching staff and Chair of the Clinical Forum. He also works as a probation officer in London, supervising high- and very high-risk violent and sexual offenders in a community-based public protection team. He has a particular interest in and experience of assessing and working with violent men from an attachment theory and research perspective. He is a member of the International Attachment Network and the International Association for Forensic Psychotherapy. He has contributed papers to *Violent Children and Adolescents: Asking the Question Why*, G. Boswell (ed.); to the *Journal of Attachment and Human Development*, H. Steele (ed.); and to *A Matter of Security: The Application of Attachment Theory to Forensic Psychiatry and Psychotherapy*, F. Pfäfflin and G. Adshead (eds).

Robert Royston has been a member of the London Centre for Psychotherapy since 1978 and is in full-time private practice. He became a training therapist in 1985 for the LCP. He supervises trainee therapists and lectures and conducts seminars on the LCP training course and on the Foundation for Psychotherapy and Counselling post-qualifications courses. He has published papers on cognitive dysfunction and narcissism in the *British Journal of Psychotherapy*; has a chapter in *Sexuality: Psychoanalytic Perspectives* (Brunner-Routledge), a chapter on self-psychology in '*Who am? The Ego and the Self in Psychoanalysis*' (Rebus Press) and a chapter on psychoanalytic technique in *Ideas in Practice* (Karnac).

Stanley Ruszczynski is a Consultant Adult Psychotherapist and Clinical Director of the Portman Clinic (Tavistock and Portman NHS Trust, London), an outpatient forensic psychotherapy clinic. He is a Senior Member of the British Association of Psychotherapists and a Direct Member of the International Psychoanalytic Association. He is a full member of the Society of Couple Psychoanalytic Psychotherapists and was previously a senior clinician at the Tavistock Marital Studies Institute and held the positions of Deputy Director and both Clinical and Training Co-ordinator. He is in private practice as a psychoanalytic psychotherapist. He has edited and co-edited five books (including *Instrusiveness and Intimacy in the Couple* (Karnac 1995), *Psychoanalytic Psychotherapy in the Kleinian Tradition* (Karnac 1999) and *Lectures of Violence, Perversion and Delinquency* (Karnac 2006)) and is the author of over 20 book chapters and journal articles. He is past Joint Editor of the *Journal of the British Association of Psychotherapists*.

Mary Thomas originally trained as an artist and, subsequently as a psychodynamic counsellor and psychoanalytic psychotherapist at WPF. She has worked in the NHS, the voluntary sector and teaches and supervises at WPF Kensington. She is a psychoanalytic psychotherapy member of FPC and has a private practice in London. She contributed a chapter to *Through the Looking Glass: Creativity in Supervision*, in C. Driver and E. Martin (eds) *Supervision and the Analytic Attitude* (Whurr 2005).

John Woods is a member of the Association of Child Psychotherapists and the British Association of Psychotherapists. He began professional life as a schoolteacher, first in a comprehensive secondary school and then in special education for 'maladjusted' children. He returned to special education after training as a child and adolescent psychotherapist. From there he went on to work with inpatients at the Cassel Hospital, specialising in the treatment of young people who self-harm. He is the author of *Boys Who Have Abused*, a play, *The End of Abuse* and several papers on clinical work in the context of educational and residential settings. Currently he is a psychotherapist at the Portman Clinic and in private practice.

Acknowledgements

This publication began as a series of lectures and seminars on aggression and destructiveness (theoretical and clinical perspectives) for professional members of the Foundation for Psychotherapy and Counselling (WPF). Some of the chapters are based on the lectures given, others were written by course participants and others fill gaps in the lecture programmes. I want to thank my friend and colleague Gill Bannister and all those FPC members who participated in these courses and contributed their ideas and rich case material to our discussions.

Every speaker on the lecture programmes contributed to my introductory chapter, 'Making sense of aggression and destructiveness', from their lectures and their recommended reading. In addition to the contributors to this publication, thanks are due to Rosine Jozef-Perelberg, Sira Dermen, Mary Twyman, Cleo Van Velson, Anne Zachary, Carlos Fishman, Rosemary Davies, David Morgan and Caroline Garland. In particular, I relied heavily on Rosine Perelberg's excellent and extensive bibliography in the review of the literature she supplies in her book *Psychoanalytic Understanding of Violence and Suicide*. I am also very grateful for the generous support and help given by to me by David Black, Susan Budd and Jospehine Klein with the writing and editing of my chapters.

An account of the healthy development of aggression was essential for this collection of papers. Marianne Parsons' chapter (p. 41) is also to be published by Karnac in David Morgan and Stanley Ruszczcynski's, *Clinical Lectures in Delinquency, Perversion and Violence*.

My thanks to Sybil del Strother who combined her skills as a psychotherapist and indexer to produce the index for this book. Also my thanks to Andrew Harvey for the thought and work he put into creating possible covers for the book.

I am especially indebted to Dorothy Lloyd-Owen for her support and help as consultant in planning the two course programmes; for her contributions to both courses; for her feedback on early drafts of my chapters in this book; and, most of all, for her supervision of my clinical work, which has enabled me to better understand and work with my own patients' destructiveness and underlying anxieties.

Lastly, and most importantly, my thanks to Michael Lamprell for his forbearance, support and encouragement throughout this lengthy project.

Part I

Mapping the terrain

Chapter 1

Making sense of aggression, destructiveness and violence

Celia Harding

Now and then an act of violence explodes into our lives and we are shockingly reminded of the human capacity for destructiveness. At that moment our reality feels violated and fragmented. 'Who is responsible?' 'When will justice be done?' 'How can it be prevented in future?' Making sense of the trauma may feel like acquiescing to the atrocity, even excusing it. Violence begets violence we know. Yet the violated mind is incapable of the thoughtful understanding that could contain our destructive reactions. Unable to think, we violently repudiate the violent act: terrorists fly aircraft into the Twin Towers and war is declared on the 'axis of evil'; a child is found dead and public outrage is violently unleashed on paedophiles; brutal murders activate demands to reinstate the death penalty. All too often the tragedy is seen as the product of an evil rather than disordered mind. Our fear of human violent and destructive capabilities paradoxically prompts us to react punitively, destructively.

This book contributes to the attempt to make sense of human aggression, destructiveness and violence perpetrated against the self, others and reality. After defining aggression, destructiveness and violence this introductory chapter outlines some of the psychoanalytic theories of aggression and explores the roots of aggression and its pathological development into destructiveness and violence; its use to disguise vulnerability and conversely, the disguises we adopt to hide, while expressing, our aggressive impulses. It ends with an exploration of some of the technical and clinical dilemmas that destructiveness may present in psychotherapy.

Defining aggression, destructiveness and violence

The *Collins Concise Dictionary* defines aggression as an attack, a harmful action, an offensive activity, a hostile or destructive mental attitude. In everyday parlance also, 'aggression' usually refers to its destructive aspect, overlooking its necessary and positive functions. In contemporary idiom 'aggressive' is sometimes used more positively to mean forceful and compelling.

Laplanche and Pontalis define aggression psychoanalytically as follows:

> Tendency or cluster of tendencies finding expression in real or phantasy behaviour intended to harm other people, or to destroy, humiliate or constrain them, etc. Violent, destructive motor action is not the only form that aggressiveness can take: indeed there is no kind of behaviour that may not have an aggressive function, be it negative – the refusal to lend assistance, for example – or positive; be it symbolic (e.g. irony) or actually carried out.
>
> (1983: 17)

Aggression is most recognisable in violence, its rawest manifestation being 'destructive motor action'. Glasser conforms to this distinction in his definition: 'violence involves bodies of both perpetrator and victim and may thus be defined as a bodily response with the intended infliction of bodily harm on another person' (Waller 1970, in Glasser 1998: 887). Perelberg (2004) extends this definition to include enactments of violent mental representations and phantasies. In particular, she suggests that the violent person is enacting a phantasy that they were conceived in a violent parental coupling (1999). Campbell (1995) regards suicidal acts as enactments of phantasised attacks on mother's body.

Psychoanalysis detects aggression where it is not immediately apparent. Aggression, like sexuality, is subject to social disapproval and constraints, and is therefore repressed and expressed in many disguises. Unconscious aggressive processes find expression in extraordinarily versatile forms. Aggression can serve many psychic functions and needs. Hence, Winnicott (1950–55) and Edgcumbe and Sandler (1974) argue that aggression is identified by intention or the underlying phantasy:

> In total psychology, being stolen from is the same as stealing and is equally aggressive. Being weak is as aggressive as the attack of the strong on the weak. Murder and suicide are fundamentally the same thing . . . possession is as aggressive as is greedy acquisition.
>
> (Winnicott 1950–55: 204)

Psychoanalysis also recognises healthy aggression. Parsons, in Chapter 3, shows how aggression promotes ego development and an active engagement with reality. In relationships, aggression is an essential ingredient of self-assertion and autonomy (Holmes 2001).

Theories of aggression

The singular contribution of psychoanalysis is that it was the first science to conceptualise aggression as an intrinsic part of our psychic structure and hence something to be accepted and not run away from.

While other theorists tended to look on aggression as an aberration and sought ways of combating it . . . Sigmund Freud firmly included aggressive behaviour within the psychosexual framework of the human being.

(Akbar 1993: 119)

Freud originally privileged sexuality but he came to recognise that aggression played a vital role in assisting the male to overcome the female's resistance to his sexual advances (1905). Fifteen years later Freud proposed that human nature included purely aggressive impulses derived from a destructive death instinct (1920). Between these two points, Freud came to identify a range of facets of human aggression. He understood that healthy aggression, facilitating the progress of the sexual instinct, could be perverted into sadism (1905). He identified hatred in the ego's repudiation of, and destructive impulses towards, unpleasurable and painful experiences. This hatred of an offensive 'other', threatening a sense of well-being, was attributed to a self-preservation instinct (1915a). Later, Freud reinforced his view of aggression as a reaction to external, as well as internal, experiences by proposing that aggression is a primary response to loss (1917). By loss he meant actual losses of loved and hated figures and emotional losses, especially narcissistic injuries to the self. In this progression (Nagera 1981), we can see aggression gradually emerging from sexuality until it is recognised as a primary facet of human nature that must be combined with, and bound by, love in order to realise its creative potentials and keep its destructive potentials in check.

Freud's successors have drawn on his insights and provided a range of theories that emphasise different aspects and functions of aggression. In particular, aggression in the service of individuation and development, self-preservation and as an inevitable part of the ambivalence we feel towards our objects. Finally, Freud came to the concept of an independent destructive drive in the 'death instinct'.

Healthy aggression

Freud recognised that we need aggression to grasp life, pursue it, master it, create it, live it. Even when he adamantly denied an independent aggressive drive he regarded aggression as an essential resource for the sexual and self-preservative instincts (1909: 140f). This early position sowed the seeds for understanding the constructive aspects of aggression. Aggression is the impetus for psychic development and integration, for independence and autonomy, for agency and mastery of the environment, for physical movement and defensive action (Freud, A. 1949; Hartmann, Kris, & Loewenstein 1949; Loewenstein 1972). Parens (1973) postulated a non-destructive aggressive current, apparent from the earliest months of life, in the baby's 'inner drivenness' to explore, tenaciously engage with and master its internal and external worlds. Aggression facilitates separation from mother and the child's individuation, contributing to the child's attachments, explorations, recoveries and learning (Solnit 1972).

Winnicott (1950–55) regarded aggression originally as synonymous with activity, essentially life generating. With time and development, love and aggression are differentiated. Children establish a sense of self as distinct from an other, and a sense of inner and outer reality, through attacking their loved ones and discovering that their attacks are survivable. If their attacks are not survived, or if their guilt is overwhelming, they are liable to inhibit their vigorous and aggressive initiatives towards others and their world, at the expense of social activity and self-development. In Chapter 3, Parsons gives a detailed account of the development of healthy aggression.

Self-preservation

In 1915 Freud assigned aggression to the self-preservative instincts, expressed particularly in a hatred of 'not-me'. Anything alien that violates the protective stimulus barrier is repudiated as a threat to psychic equilibrium. The idea of aggression in the service of self-preservation is the basis for understanding aggression provoked by a perception that the self and identity is under threat from internal or external dangers.

In Chapter 6, Ruszczynski elaborates, with vivid case illustrations, Glasser's concepts of self-preservative aggression and the core complex. Self-preservative aggression aims 'to remove or negate any element which stands between the individual and the meeting of his needs or his survival' (Glasser 1996: 281). Anything that disturbs psychic equilibrium or threatens identity may provoke self-preservative aggression. Increasing mental disturbance is accompanied by mounting aggression. Glasser contrasts self-preservative aggression and sadism. People with a precarious sense of self are convinced that their longings for intimacy will compromise their psychic existence. A longing for closeness induces murderous rage toward the person they yearn for. But being alone also threatens their fragile sense of self: eliminating the threatening person means eliminating the person they need. They resolve this dilemma by sexualising their self-preservative aggression, turning it into sadism, thereby converting the wish to destroy into the wish to control and hurt. The consequent sado-masochistic relationship protects them from the threat of intimacy while sustaining an intense relationship at a safe distance, neither too close nor too far away. The anxieties associated with either intimacy or abandonment are eroticised and turned from murderous rage into excitement.

Threats to an unstable identity often lead to violent behaviour (Glasser 1998: 889). Perelberg (1999) suggests that violence may serve an organising function when people feel that their identity is liable to fragment or when they fear they may become helpless. This may particularly apply to men for whom being masculine means 'not-feminine', when femininity is equated with vulnerability and dependency (Denman 2003: 151f). Violent behaviour may seem to promise a 'quick fix' for a failing sense of masculinity, for example, by using a gun as 'an accessory'. Women also may resort to violent behaviour to counteract despised and dangerous feelings of vulnerability and dependency and the attendant risk of engulfment (Perelberg 1999). Alternatively, men and woman may erotise their aggressive antidote to vulnerability, turning it into powerful sexual seductiveness.

Self-preservative destructiveness also takes the form of attacks against the self when the self is felt to be at risk of exposure to re-traumatising experiences. Mollon (2002), for example, explores the impact of gross violations to the self when the 'psychological environment' has been experienced as 'intent on psychic murder – wanting to do away with the child's actual self and replace it with an alternative preferred version' (2002: 53). When children's needs and initiatives are repeatedly rejected by a person on whom they rely, they come to regard their own feelings, especially vulnerability and the need for others, as dangerous. One solution is to identify with the aggressor and kill off their own feelings and needs, destroying their emotional life before they are destroyed emotionally. Intimacy can similarly be eliminated as a potential threat. From a Jungian perspective, Kalsched (1996) describes how any sign of vulnerability may induce a self-destructive attack, in an attempt to protect the self from violation. Rather than trust people in intimate relationships, and risk being re-traumatised by them, the traumatised self elects to destroy its own neediness and vulnerability. 'Aggressive, destructive energies – ordinarily available for reality-adaptation and for healthy defence against toxic not-self objects – are directed back into the inner world' (Kalsched 1996: 19). Examples of aggression that has been deployed for survival at the expense of development are given by Renn in Chapter 4, Harding in Chapter 8, Christie in Chapter 10, Kleimberg in Chapter 11, and Thomas in Chapter 14.

Reaction to loss and fear of loss

Freud (1917) suggests that people cannot mourn their loved objects until they have come to terms with their unresolved hatred towards them. Meanwhile, the ego identifies with loved aspects of the lost one and the superego absorbs the hostility towards the lost object and directs it onto the ego. This was the point of departure for theories of destructive aggression understood as reactions to a lost, disappointing or failing object, originally experienced in an actual, external relationship and subsequently internalised and represented in the mind. Kleimberg, in Chapter 11, and Lucas, in Chapter 12, illustrate the pervasive and corrosive impact of installing the hostile aspect of the relationship in the mind.

The view that aggression is a reaction to separation and loss is illustrated by Fairbairn (1952). He considers the mind to be structured as a network of internalised relationships with the primary caregiver. Separation from mother activates the dependent infant's frustrated aggression and promotes an internalisation of the frustrating relationships with her (1952: 17f, 54f, 109). The infant fears that its neediness, erotic longings and frustrated rage will jeopardise its necessary relationship with mother. Aggression is mobilised to subdue these dangerous feelings, thus averting the catastrophic consequences of mother's rejection (1952: 173). The infant attempts to control both the bad, frustrating mother and his hatred of her, by internalising these aspects of their relationship; in this way the infant can appear to preserve the external mother as loved, available and satisfying. This manoeuvre relocates the problem from the external relationship into the mind, where both the object and the ego are split into subsidiary internal relationships. The mother is split into an exciting figure desired by a libidinal needy ego and a frustrating, rejecting figure engaged with an anti-libidinal ego. The central ego mobilises aggression to repress both these painful relationships. By internalising and repressing her exciting and rejecting aspects, the relationship with the external mother is preserved as idealised, beyond reproach and longing (1952: 136).

In sum, Fairbairn regards the child's aggression as a primary instinct that is mobilised when mother frustrates libidinal needs. Infants direct their aggression inwards in a misguided attempt to keep the relationship with the mother aggression-free and therefore protected from rejection. The price of keeping the relationship with mother safe from both instinctual loving and aggressive feelings is the establishment of internal relationships that deploy aggressive energies to attack and subdue vulnerability, longing and neediness.

In Chapter 4, Renn elaborates Bowlby's theories, also based on understanding aggression as a reaction to separation from, and loss of, an attachment figure. In attachment theory, our need for others has a biological basis. We require reliable proximity to our attachment figures for physical survival and by extension we develop an adaptive physiological, emotional and cognitive system to explore the world and make new attachments throughout life (DeZulueta 1993; Fonagy 2001; Holmes 1993). The infant keeps its attachment figures close by with a repertoire of attachment behaviours. Angry protest when the attachment figure leaves or returns discourages separations. Bowlby, and the theorists developing his work, have understood destructive aggression as an extension of natural angry protests at the loss or absence of attachment figures, particularly when these losses have not been mediated by mitigating circumstances (Holmes 1993).

Attachment theorists see the child's internalised attachments as 'internal working models' of relationships. Renn describes how children with internal working models based on secure relationships expect responsiveness from their caregivers and are confident of being loved and wanted. Conversely, when the internal working models are based on attachments with an unreliable, unresponsive, frightened and/or frightening caregiver the child is likely to see itself as unwanted, unlovable and unworthy. Insecurely attached children become locked into their attachment with their caregiver internally and externally, neither able to separate from, nor change the basis of, their attachment (Carvalho 2002: 167).

Renn also argues that secure attachments are the necessary context for the development of affect regulation, impulse control, empathy, mentalisation and, therefore, interpersonal competence (Fonagy 2001). Without the empathic attunement of a secure attachment, children cannot develop the mental capacities necessary to regulate and make sense of losses and the aggression they evoke. Instead, the internal working models reproduce in the mind the way 'of regulating (or not) one's affects as one's primary caregiver does: one behaves towards one's emotions as they do and did and indeed as one fantasises them to do and to have done' (Carvalho 2002: 167).

Renn shows clearly how people without the capacity to regulate their feelings are prone to express their strong emotions in primitive ways such as self-harm and violence towards others. He demonstrates how destructive and violent reactions to vulnerability and loss frequently indicate lost or damaged attachments earlier in life (see also DeZulueta 1993; Fonagy 2001; Holmes 1993). People who are unable to empathise with losses because they are reminded of their own overwhelming pain, are likely to attack rather than respect vulnerability, and their working models of relationships are likely to be organised on the basis of victim and perpetrator (Carvalho 2002; DeZulueta 1993). Woods, in Chapter 9, explores this dynamic in the example of bullies and their victims.

The death instinct

Freud's arrival at his concept of the death instinct (1920) revealed aggression as an end in itself rather than a means to an end (Schmidt-Hellerau 2002: 1271). The idea of the death instinct emerged from Freud's struggle to understand the ubiquitous human compulsion to repeat painful experiences (Black 2001; Laplanche & Pontalis 1983). Freud proposed that a struggle between the life instincts to connect and integrate and the death instincts to dissolve and destroy, operates at every level of our biological and psychological being. Resulting fusions and defusions of the life and death instincts determine the relative strength and weakness of impulses to grow and develop or stagnate and degenerate. The death instinct is directed at the self and operates invisibly and unhindered when it is not bound by life forces. Observable destructiveness derives from the death instinct and is directed outwards for self-preservation. In the internal world, aggression is expressed as sadism towards the self and experienced as guilt. Freud understood a person's guilt as proportionate to the aggression they redirected from other people back onto themselves, absorbed into the superego and converted into sadistic attacks on the ego (1930). Similarly in melancholia, as Lucas movingly shows in Chapter 12, an excessively harsh superego turns against the lost object in the ego with the force of 'the pure culture of the death instinct' (1923).

Melanie Klein and her followers saw the death instinct as a primary determinant of psychic development (see King & Steiner 1991). Klein concluded that the inhibitions of the children she analysed stemmed from their anxieties about their aggressive impulses. Klein equated the death instinct with sadism expressed through an archaic superego (Hinshelwood 1991: 48). In her view, the death instinct underlies the infant's aggressive impulses and phantasies towards the good breast from birth and is liable to undermine the benign and satisfying experiences offered by the good mother. In the 'paranoid-schizoid position', infants manage their aggression by attributing it to the bad breast, kept separate from their nurturing experiences with the good breast (Klein 1946). The 'depressive position' is achieved when good and bad breast are seen as aspects of the same person, capable of surviving the infant's sadism and envy and thus enabling a good object to be introjected and loving feelings to modify destructive impulses (Klein 1935).

The death instinct, according to Kleinian theory, is part of the human constitution and operative from birth. In Chapters 12 and 13, Lucas and Amos show the pervasively destructive influence of the death instinct on internal and external relationships. In particular, hostility is directed towards the needy libidinal self and objects offering to meet those needs. Conversely, omnipotent positions in internal and external relationships are idealised as beyond pain, guilt and vulnerability. These internal relations are the basis for psychotic and pathological organisations of the mind aimed at maintaining idealised destructiveness and keeping need and vulnerability under constant attack (Rosenfeld 1971; Steiner 1993).

By proposing the death instinct as central to psychic development, Kleinian theory challenged the 'privilege' that psychoanalysis had accorded to libido (King & Steiner 1991: 513). A theoretical distinction emerged between those following Klein, who believed that a tendency to self- and object-destructiveness emanated from an overbearing destructive instinct fuelled by the death instinct (illustrated by Lucas in Chapter 12 and Amos in Chapter 13) and those following Anna Freud, who believed that it was failures in libidinal development that led to overactive destructiveness (illustrated by Parsons in Chapter 3).

The concept of the death instinct has remained contentious in psychoanalysis. Black (2001) outlines some formidable theoretical difficulties inherent in the theory of the death drive. He argues that in retrospect it can be regarded as 'a detour' on the way to Freud's identification of an independent destructive drive. Lucas, conversely, represents the view (Chapter 12) that psychotic states of mind confirm the reality of the death instinct. In contrast, Royston (Chapter 2) argues that states of acute vulnerability lie behind an apparent drive towards inertia.

An integrated theory of aggression

As Schmidt-Hellerau elegantly points out, each theory highlights an important aspect of human aggression:

> Hardly anyone would dispute that aggression is something 'driven', inherent in human nature (that is, biogenetically based); it is equally correct to say that it arises in response to frustration and danger and within object relationships; and it is virtually self-evident that, besides hostile (malignant) aggression, there is also useful (benign) aggression.
>
> (2002: 1270)

Mitchell (1993) comes close to offering a theory of aggression that integrates the features identified by Freud. The exception, in his view is constructive assertiveness (1993: 362), which he sees as deriving from a different source in our psychology:

> From the drive theory side comes the notion that aggression is biologically based, physiologically powerful, and universal, playing an inevitable and central dynamic role in the generation of experience and the shaping of the self. From the nondrive theory side comes the notion that aggression is a response to endangerment within the personally designed subjective world, not a pre-psychological push looking for a reason.
>
> (1993: 373)

Mitchell sees aggression as a central organiser of our sense of self. As a 'pre-wired potential' of our biology, aggression arises as part of our nature. Aggression, like sexual desire, has a power derived from its physiological base. When strong aggressive reactions have not been 'mentalised' they seem to take us over:

> Intense anger is arresting and pre-emptive. When unintegrated, it can shatter and diffuse other concerns and intentions; its physiological power can disorganise mental states. When integrated, it can generate and energise other motives and actions. Aggression, like sexuality, often provides the juice that potentiates and embellishes experience.
>
> (Mitchell 1993: 371)

Aggression acquires personal meanings for each individual as their aggressive impulses emerge and take shape in the context of their relationships. In other words, our destructive feelings acquire meanings from the ways others evoke, receive and understand our aggressive initiatives and responses. Destructiveness is evoked when the sense of self feels endangered. In particular, the prolonged dependency of human beings on others during infancy inclines us to experience responsive failures as threats to our psychological, and sometimes physiological, survival throughout life (Mitchell 1993).

Coming to terms with aggression

Developmental roots

Infants engage with the world using a repertoire of emotional resources including aggression. In favourable circumstances, the world provides them with the conditions they need to utilise their aggression for survival, self-assertion and creativity rather than destructiveness. In the first instance, as Parsons describes in Chapter 3, infants need an empathic and emotionally available mother capable of receiving and containing her baby's loving and aggressive impulses. Fortunate infants discover in the mother a consistent and reliable empathic responsiveness at times when they are overwhelmed by their needs and feelings. As children gradually internalise experiences of empathically responsive figures as good objects to turn to in states of helplessness and distress, they learn that it is safe to be vulnerable in the presence of a protective object (Parsons & Dermen 1999). Good internal objects contain and integrate with loving feelings, the powerful feelings of aggression aroused by threatening experiences. When feelings can be contained and thought about by a protective object the child can begin to symbolise and process their feelings mentally (Garland 2002; Segal 1957).

In psychoanalysis, the containing qualities of empathic responsiveness to the infant, combined with protectiveness from external impingements, is represented as the maternal function. A mother's maternal function is compromised when her child's emotional states are experienced as a threat to her own psychic equilibrium. In Chapter 10, Christie gives examples of mothers who were not psychically available to attend to their children's emotional needs: unable to contain their own feelings these mothers turned to their children to meet their needs. In such circumstances, a child is liable to grow up with a precarious sense of self and a reservoir of rage and hatred, lacking the mental capacities to manage these powerful emotions. Without an understanding and protective internal object to turn to, or the mental processes to symbolise their aggression, the endangered self resorts to destructive defensive measures. This consequence is illustrated by Harding (Chapter 8), Christie (Chapter 10) and Kleimberg (Chapter 11), who give case examples of women who had not internalised protective, empathic figures to contain their aggressive states of mind. Instead, these women managed their aggression destructively by turning it against their own needs and wishes.

The maternal function in the child's development is complemented by the paternal function of separation and individuation, represented in psychoanalysis as the role of the father. Children need a 'third' in their lives to help them to separate from mother and to mediate the demands of external reality. When the father intervenes in the relationship between mother and child to 'reclaim' his wife and establish a relationship of his own with his child (Campbell 1995), he offers the child 'a way out' of an exclusive dependence on mother. In order to develop an independent identity, the child needs help to separate from mother and encouragement to express their independent strivings, often in the form of angry protests. Failure to achieve this separation jeopardises the child's developing sense of self and makes it difficult later in life to establish either intimate relationships with, or autonomy from, others (Glasser 1992; Holmes 2001). Without a consistent and reliable father to turn to as an alternative and different source of support and protection, estrangement from mother is liable to be experienced as abandonment without a container (Carvalho 2002), propelling the child back to the symbiotic relationship with mother (Leowald 1951). As alternative figures to turn to, fathers offer children different ways of seeing mother, themselves, and their relationship with mother. The child is released from their symbiotic relationship with mother by seeing that there is more than one way to interact with her (Fonagy & Target 1995). In this observing position (Britton 1989), children can reflect on and think about their experiences with mother rather than be immersed in, and overwhelmed by, them. Therefore as Kleimberg shows (Chapter 11) the paternal function provides the mental space for thought and symbolisation enabling aggressive feelings to be managed and expressed creatively rather than internalised destructively.

In Chapter 5, Harrison describes how boys with violent fathers face a dilemma about how to manage their aggressive feelings. In favourable circumstances, young boys identify with fathers who have protected and supported their strivings to become independent of mother (Leowald 1951) and helped them to manage their longings for an exclusive union with mother (Campbell 1995). This identification helps the child to experience father's presentation of the 'facts of life' (see Ruszczynski, Chapter 6) as more supportive than punishing (Leowald 1951). Identifying with a supportive and protective father provides the boy with the basis to develop a secure masculine identity (Glasser 1992). However, when the father is violent, emotionally and especially physically, identification with father exposes the child to frightening levels of unmanageable aggression. The young boy's attempts to become independent of mother are hampered because father is unavailable as a protective supportive object and because his aggression feels too alarming to use in the service of self-assertion. The boy's aggression, particularly self-preservative aggression, is liable to violently erupt when he perceives a threat to his identity because he lacks the capacity to distance himself in more sophisticated and imaginative ways. Harrison describes the regressive defences her patient developed to sustain a semblance of identity without the aid of the aggression he equated with his father's violence.

Aggression in disguise and as disguise

We find ways to manage our destructive impulses with the psychic and physical resources at our disposal. These solutions may be heavily disguised to make them acceptable to our disapproving loved objects and, in turn, to our superegos. The contributors to this book illustrate examples of aggression in disguise and as disguise. For example, Kleimberg (Chapter 11) shows how aggression can be disguised by the hopelessness and despair of depression. Harrison (Chapter 5), and Rusczcynski (Chapter 6) show how sexual excitement may perversely disguise underlying hatred and violence. Harding (Chapter 8) and Christie (Chapter 10) illustrate how the role of innocent victim can disguise unprocessed rage and destructiveness from traumatic experiences. Lucas (Chapter 12) shows how denial and rationalisation in psychosis conceal massive attacks on reality and the self. Conversely, the endangered self, weakened by the deficient containment of its primary objects may disguise itself in destructive ways. This is illustrated by Mann (Chapter 7) in his exploration of the hatred of the misanthropist; by Renn (Chapter 4) who gives examples of physical violence defending against vulnerability; by Woods (Chapter 9) who explores the victim underlying the bully and by Royston (Chapter 2), Amos (Chapter 13), and Thomas (Chapter 14) in their examples of destructive attacks on therapy.

As Ruszczynski explains in Chapter 6, without the psychic means to contain overwhelming states of mind, the self becomes overwhelmed by pain, loss or terror, the capacity to mentalise feelings collapses and the person becomes liable to resort to action as a concrete form of containment. Destructiveness that cannot be processed mentally has to be evacuated and/or enacted. There are broadly three solutions to the problem of containment when the capacity for symbolisation collapses (Garland 2002):

1   People may identify with their designated aggressor and turn their passive experience of helplessness into active perpetration of what was done to them. This defence may lead to depressed or vengeful states of mind as shown by Kleimberg in Chapter 11, Harding in Chapter 8, Christie in Chapter 10, Woods in Chapter 9, and Thomas in Chapter 14.

2   People may eroticise their overwhelming experiences and turn pain, anxiety and rage into excitement and adopt perverse defences and solutions as shown by Rusczcynski in Chapter 6 and Harrison in Chapter 5.

3   Those with highly unstable identities react violently when they feel psychically threatened. In extremity, the endangered self resorts to psychotic functioning by attacking the perceptual capacities (Segal 1957, 1986). Psychic pain may be experienced and expressed bodily when it cannot be processed psychically (Fonagy & Target 1995). Uncontainable psychic pain may be projected into a victim who may be violently attacked and/or murdered or the psychic pain may be introjected into the body as in self-harm or suicide (Anderson 1997; Bell 2000; Sohn 1997; Williams 1995). These violent solutions are illustrated by Renn in Chapter 4, Ruszczynski in Chapter 6 and Lucas in Chapter 13.

Working with destructiveness in the clinical situation

Aggression is an essential ingredient in psychotherapy. Integrated aggression energises engagement with the therapist in self-assertion and contributes perseverance and determination to the therapeutic alliance. Unintegrated aggression may disrupt the progress of therapy, preventing or disturbing engagement with the therapist. The psychotherapeutic relationship offers patients an opportunity to integrate their aggression more satisfactorily so it may become a useful resource, rather than a disruptive factor, in their mental and relational economy. However, the ego strength required to mentally process powerful aggressive and sexual impulses is only achieved through containing destabilising feelings. Therapists fulfil the dual functions of maternal containing and paternal separating and differentiating for their patients until the patient has internalised these capacities for themselves, through symbolic thought rather than re-action (Garland 2002; Segal 1957).

Freud recognised the undermining influence of unintegrated aggression in resistances to therapy (Laplanche & Pontalis 1983). Having identified the destructive instinct, he detected its role in impeding the progress of recovery in psychotherapy:

> No stronger impression arises from the resistances during the work of analysis than of there being a force which is defending itself by every possible means against recovery and which is absolutely resolved to hold onto illness and suffering.
>
> (1937: 243)

Part of the therapist's task is to understand the patient's shifting motives for tenaciously holding onto their suffering. Suffering may, for example, appease a cruel and unforgiving superego (Glasser 1986, 1992); gain pleasure from triumphing over the therapist and the needy part of the self (Feldman 2000); be chosen as a lesser evil to facing the dreaded pain of losing the good object (Bell 2000) or secure base (Holmes 2001) or guilt for damage done (Anderson 1997; Steiner 1993).

Freud recognised that ego weaknesses make it difficult to manage aggressive impulses constructively. He attributed ego weakness to two main factors: the strength of the destructive instinct, and a traumatised ego inadequately protected by the stimulus barrier and overwhelmed by experiences from internal or/and external sources (Freud 1937). Psychoanalytic opinions acknowledge the interactive influence of both factors undermining the ego's capacity to integrate and regulate aggression. However, opinions tend to divide between those emphasising the strength of the destructive instinct (e.g. Feldman 2000; Hinshelwood 1991; King & Steiner 1991; Klein 1946, 1957; Segal 1957, 1986) and those emphasising reactions to environmental experiences, in particular the impact of trauma, deprivation and failures of maternal containment (e.g. DeZulueta 1993; Fairbairn 1952; Fonagy 2001; Fonagy & Target 1995; Kalsched 1996; Mollon 1998, 2002). In Chapter 2, Royston thoroughly and elegantly explores the implications of this theoretical debate for understanding the progress of clinical work.

Therapists know that what they say or become for the patient may be experienced as threatening (Parsons & Dermen 1999). The structure of the therapeutic relationship may expose patients to their own limitations and activate their frustrated rage and hatred. The therapeutic relationship, particularly the therapist's empathy and compassion, makes patients more aware of their needs and vulnerabilities provoking a defensive reaction when these are felt to endanger the self (Fonagy & Target 1995). Glasser offers a catalogue of such external and internal threats liable to provoke self-protective destructive or violent reactions. Experiences perceived as endangering the patient's gender identity, provoking frustration, disempowerment or humiliation, insulting an ideal self, undermining self-esteem. The patient may feel at risk of unbearable confusion, disintegration or remorseless castigation by a tyrannical, sadistic superego (Glasser 1998: 889).

Psychic change inevitably destabilises the patient's psychic equilibrium. But when the capacity to symbolise and reflect on feelings is unstable or non-existent, the patient risks reliving threatening feelings and relationships, and becoming re-traumatised (Kalsched 1996). The patient's trust in the therapist, to be a reliable good object/secure base with whom it feels safe to be vulnerable and needy, has to be established and re-established over and over again. 'It is only once that [therapeutic] bond is formed that the controlled turbulence and challenge needed for new meanings to emerge can hope to succeed' (Holmes 2001: 46). In Chapter 13, Amos gives examples of such psychic destabilisation from the perspective of the equilibrium between the life and death instincts.

Therapy may constellate a number of double binds for the patient, evoking feelings of helplessness and rage. For example, the patient's need to rely on the therapist may re-expose them to disappointments, betrayals, neglects experienced in past dependent relationships. Their longings for closeness may threaten psychic extinction, but their longings for separateness and independence threaten abandonment (Glasser 1996). The therapist's empathic understanding may be experienced as the presence of an engulfing mother threatening the patient's sense of self and evoking self-preservative rage to create a distance from the threatening therapist (Glasser 1992; Perelberg 1999, 2004). The therapist's separating and differentiating functions, in the form of interpretation and maintaining the analytic frame, may evoke rage and alarm that this rage could escalate into violence provoking regression to a fusional state (Perelberg 1999, 2004). The patient's desperation to engage with life, as represented by the therapy, may evoke pain beyond endurance and, as Amos understands it in Chapter 13, may provoke a deadly backlash. The prospect of possession means having to face the risk of loss, that is to say, death (Freud 1915b): 'It is better to have loved and lost than never to have loved at all' only rings true for those with considerable ego strength. This dilemma is faced at every session where the end is presaged in its beginning, at breaks between sessions, at holiday breaks and with the fact of life that all good things come to an end, including the therapeutic relationship. Connecting with the pain of loss exposes the patient to guilt and grief for the damage they have inflicted on their good objects (Anderson 1997; Steiner 1994) and the life they have hitherto not lived (Kalsched 1996).

Destructive impulses rarely appear in the consulting room in the form of overt physical violence because when a threat to psychic equilibrium is too overwhelming to be thought, the patient can literally take flight or project the intolerable state of mind into the therapist (see, for example, Thomas Chapter 14). Threats may be reacted to actively or passively, in spontaneous outbursts or in organised ways. As in everyday life (p. 14f) there are broadly three types of solution to the problem of disposing of and expressing helpless rage when experiences beyond the ego's capacities arise in the therapeutic relationship (Garland 2002). First, patients may turn their perceived helplessness into active identification with the aggressor. The aggressor may be the lost, disappointing or traumatising object represented in an internal relationship and reincarnated with the therapist. Patients may perceive their therapist as mistreating them and exploiting their trust. This shifts the passive vulnerable patient into the powerful position of a victim with a valid grievance justly attacking the therapist. Second, patients may eroticise the rage induced by their helplessness and dependency on the therapist. They may attempt to turn the therapeutic relationship into a sexual seduction (Kernberg 1995: 115). Or patients may convert the therapeutic relationship into a sado-masochistic one, where the patient feels safely in control of the therapist kept at a safe distance, not too close and not too far. Third, the self in extreme danger resorts to psychotic solutions. A psychotic part of the mind appropriates the mental apparatus and attacks the perception of reality and the perceiving self (Rosenfeld 1987; Segal 1986). Royston, in Chapter 2, Amos, in Chapter 13, and Thomas, in Chapter 14, give examples of patients who feel caught between the pain of life, development, and action and the pain of annihilation through fragmentation and inertia and illustrate the deadly processes that are activated in the therapeutic process. Lucas, in Chapter 12, shows how these processes may be expressed through identifying the threatening object with the body resulting in physical symptoms or suicidal thoughts or projected into an external object and murderously attacked. These solutions represent defences against less endurable suffering and may be attempts to protect good internal and external objects from harm (Bell 2000; Zetzel 1953). Garland (2002) emphasises that rage evoked by helplessness is a sign of life with a vital protective function providing a 'semblance of coherence' and psychic organisation at a point of fragmentation (2002: 210). However, when destructiveness is not psychically contained this reaction may compound the damage.

The therapist detects the expression of destructive impulses and phantasies through transference and counter-transference communications. Frequently, therapists become aware of an urgent pressure to do or say something, to act rather than think in response to the patient's projected states of mind. The pressure may be an id pressure, to let 'anything go' or a superego pressure to resort to harsh, judgmental 'easy certainties' but, in either case, the therapist is required to process the projections and then re-present the unbearable experiences in thoughtful understanding (Anderson 1997; Holmes 2001; Lloyd-Owen 2002). The therapist needs an open mind to see things from the patient's point of view (Steiner 1994) and to hold the projections until they can be understood. This containing process introduces the patient to the process of thinking about mental states (Fonagy & Target 1995; Parsons & Dermen 1999). The therapist gradually articulates the patient's underlying anxieties and dilemmas (Glasser 1992; Perelberg 1999, 2004) and shows the patient the illusory clarity of their violent or destructive solutions (Fonagy & Target 1995). Any direct interpretation of patients' aggression towards the therapist is likely to be futile and counterproductive (Fonagy & Target 1995) and may compound patient's dread that they are irredeemable and their destructiveness is uncontainable (Rosenfeld 1987; Steiner 1994). However, trust in the therapist will be jeopardised if patients perceive their therapist as defeated by, or colluding with, their destructiveness (Steiner 1994). Rosenfeld (1987) suggests that the patient's vulnerability must be carefully assessed and that it may be more helpful to interpret the patient's inertia and paralysis as fear of explosive rage, rather than focus on the destructive rage itself. Glasser defines the therapist's task as showing the patient how their ways of managing work against them. But he cautions:

Ultimately the patient may know better than we do what is his optimal solution and it has to be left to him to 'choose' how he prefers to reconcile the complex interaction of factors which make up his psychological world – indeed the analyst cannot do otherwise.

(1992: 500)

The capacity to contain destructiveness in damage-limited ways generates hope of psychic reparation (Klein 1937, 1957; Rey 1996)). Harding, in Chapter 8 shows how this may be achieved in the therapeutic relationship when a protective and containing object has been internalised and the painful process of mourning has been endured. As the patient's superego becomes less cruel and demanding of perfection and more forgiving, the ego can accept forgiveness, compromise and imperfect repair. Hope and gratitude then become possible. These are hard won and inestimable achievements.

References

Akbar, M. (1993) 'The psychoanalytic concept of aggression', *Journal of the Indian Psychoanalytical Society* 47(4): 118–28

Anderson, R. (1997) 'Putting the boot in: violent defences against depressive anxiety' in *Reason and Passion. A Celebration of the Work of Hanna Segal*, D. Bell (ed.), London: Duckworth

Bell, D. (2000) 'Who is killing what or whom? Some notes on the internal phenomenology of suicide', *Psychoanalytic Psychotherapy* 15(1): 21–37

Black, D. (2001) 'Mapping a detour: why did Freud speak of a death drive?', *British Journal of Psychotherapy* 18(2): 189–98

Britton, R. (1989) 'The missing link: parental sexuality in the Oedipus complex' in *The Oedipus Complex Today*, J. Steiner (ed.), London: Karnac

Campbell, D. (1995) 'The role of the father in a pre-suicide state', *International Journal of Psychoanalysis* 76(2): 315–23

Carvalho, R. (2002) 'Psychic retreats revisited: binding primitive destructiveness or securing the object? A matter of emphasis?', *British Journal of Psychotherapy* 19(2): 153–71

Denman, C. (2003) *Sexuality: A Biopsychosocial Approach*, Basingstoke: Palgrave Macmillan

DeZulueta, F. (1993) *From Pain to Violence. The Traumatic Roots of Destructiveness*. London: Whurr

Edgcumbe, R. and Sandler, J. (1974) 'Some comments on aggression turned against the self: a brief communication', *International Journal of Psychoanalysis* 55(3): 365–67

Fairbairn, W.R.D. (1952) *Psychoanalytic Studies of the Personality*, London and New York: Routledge

Feldman, M. (2000) 'Some views on the manifestation of the death instinct in clinical work', *International Journal of Psychoanalysis* 81(1): 53–65

Fonagy, P. (2001) *Attachment Theory and Psychoanalysis*, New York: The Other Press

Fonagy, P. and Target, M. (1995) 'Understanding the violent patient: the use of the body and the role of the father' in *Psychoanalytic Understanding Violence and Suicide*, R. Perelberg (ed.), London and New York: Routledge

Freud, A. (1949) 'Aggression in relation to emotional development: normal and pathological', *Psychoanalytic Study of the Child* 3–4: 37–42

—— (1972) 'Comments on aggression', *International Journal of Psychoanalysis* 53: 163–71

Freud, S. (1905) 'Three essays on sexuality', *Standard Edition 7*, London: Hogarth Press

—— (1909) 'Analysis of a phobia in a five year old boy', *Standard Edition 10*, London: Hogarth Press

—— (1915a) 'Instincts and their vicissitudes', *Standard Edition 14*, London: Hogarth Press

—— (1915b) 'Thoughts for the times on war and death', *Standard Edition 14*, London: Hogarth Press

—— (1917) 'Mourning and melancholia', *Standard Edition 14*, London: Hogarth Press

—— (1920) 'Beyond the pleasure principle', *Standard Edition 18*, London: Hogarth Press

—— (1923) 'The ego and the id', *Standard Edition 19*, London: Hogarth Press

—— (1930) 'Civilisation and its discontents', *Standard Edition 21*, London: Hogarth Press

—— (1937) 'Analysis terminable and interminable', *Standard Edition 23*, London: Hogarth Press

Garland, C. (2002) 'Action, identification and thought in post-traumatic states' in *Understanding Trauma: A Psychoanalytical Approach*, C. Garland (ed.), London and New York: Karnac

Glasser, M. (1986) 'Identification and its vicissitudes', *International Journal of Psychoanalysis* 67: 9–17

—— (1992) 'Problems in the psychoanalysis of certain narcissistic disorders', *International Journal of Psychoanalysis* 73: 493–502

—— (1996) 'Aggression and sadism in the perversions' in *Sexual Deviation* 3rd edition, I. Rosen (ed.), Oxford: Oxford University Press

—— (1998) 'On violence: a preliminary communication', *International Journal of Psychoanalysis* 79: 887–902

Hartmann, H., Kris, E. and Loewenstein, R.M. (1949) 'Notes on the theory of aggression', *Psychoanalytic Study of the Child* 3–4: 9–36

Hinshelwood, R.D. (1991) *A Dictionary of Kleinian Thought*, London: Free Association Books

Holmes, J. (1993) *John Bowlby and Attachment Theory*, Hove and New York: Brunner-Routledge

—— (2001) *The Search for a Secure Base. Attachment Theory and Psychotherapy*, Hove and New York: Brunner-Routledge

Hyatt-Williams, H. (1995) 'Murderousness in relationship to psychotic breakdown (madness)' in *Psychosis and Treatment*, J. Ellwood (ed.), London and Bristol, PA: Jessica Kingsley

Kalsched, D. (1996) *The Inner World of Trauma. Archetypal Defences of the Personal Spirit*, New York and London: Routledge

Kernberg, O. (1995) *Love Relations: Normality and Pathology*, New Haven, CT and London: Yale University Press

King, P. and Steiner, R. (1991) *The Freud-Klein Controversies 1941–45*, London and New York: Tavistock/Routledge

Klein, M. (1935) 'A contribution to the psychogenesis of manic depressive states', *Love, Guilt and Reparation and other Works 1921–1945*, London: Virago

—— (1937) 'Love, guilt and reparation', *Love, Guilt and Reparation and other Works 1921–1945*, London: Virago

—— (1946) 'Notes on some schizoid mechanisms', *Envy and Gratitude and Other Works*, London: Hogarth Press

—— (1957) 'Envy and gratitude', *Envy and Gratitude and Other Works*, London: Hogarth Press

Laplanche, J. and Pontalis, J.B. (1983) *The Language of Psycho-Analysis*, London: Hogarth Press

Leowald, H.W. (1951) 'Ego and reality' in *Papers on Psychoanalysis*, H.W. Leowald, New Haven, CT and London: Yale University Press

Lloyd-Owen, D. (2002) 'Supervising work where patients damage themselves and others', unpublished paper

Loewenstein, R.M. (1972) 'Panel on aggression. Panel discussion at 27th International Psychoanalytic Congress, Vienna 29th July 1971', *International Journal of Psychoanalysis* 53 13–19

Mitchell, S.A. (1993) 'Aggression and the endangered self', *Psychoanalytic Quarterly* 62(3): 351–82

Mollon, P. (1998) *Remembering Trauma*, Chichester and New York: John Wiley & Sons

—— (2002) *Shame and Jealousy: The Hidden Turmoils*, London: Karnac

Nagera, H. (ed.) (1981) *Basic Psychoanalytic Concepts on the Libido Theory*, London: Karnac

Parens, H. (1973) 'Aggression: a reconsideration', *Journal of American Psychoanalytic Association* 21(1): 34–60

Parsons, M. and Dermen, S. (1999) 'The violent child and adolescent' in *The Handbook of Child and Adolescent Psychotherapy*, M. Lanyado and A. Horne (eds), London and New York: Routledge

Perelberg, R. (1999) 'A core phantasy in violence' in *Psychoanalytic Understanding Violence and Suicide*, R. Perelberg (ed.), London and New York: Routledge

—— (2004) 'Narcissistic configurations: violence and its absence in treatment', *International Journal of Psychoanalysis* 85: 1065–79

Rey, H. (1996) 'Reparation in universals of psychoanalysis' in *The Treatment of Psychotic and Borderline States*, London: Free Association Books

Rosenfeld, H. (1971) 'A clinical approach to the psychoanalytic theory of the life and death instincts: an investigation into the aggressive aspects of narcissism' in *Melanie Klein Today: Mainly Theory*, Vol. 1, E. Bott Spillius (ed.), London and New York: Routledge

—— (1987) 'Afterthought: changing theories and techniques in analysis' in *Impasse and Interpretation*, London: Routledge

Segal, H. (1957) 'Notes on symbol formation' in *Melanie Klein Today: Mainly Theory*, E. Bott Spillius (ed.), London and New York: Routledge

—— (1986) 'On the clinical usefulness of the concept of the death instinct' in *Psychoanalysis, Literature and War: Papers 1972–95*, London and New York: Routledge

Schmidt-Hellerau, C. (2002) 'Why aggression?', *International Journal of Psychoanalysis* 83(6): 1269–89

Sohn, L. (1997) 'Unprovoked assaults: making sense of apparently random violence' in *Reason and Passion A Celebration of the Work of Hanna Segal*, D. Bell (ed.), London: Duckworth

Solnit, A.J. (1972) 'Aggression: a view of theory building in psychoanalysis', *Journal of the American Psychoanalytic Association* 20(3): 435–50

Steiner, J. (1993) *Psychic Retreats: Pathological Organisations in Psychotic, Neurotic and Borderline Patients*, London: Routledge

—— (1993) 'Problems of psychoanalytic technique: patient-centred and analyst-centred interpretations', *Psychic Retreats*, London and New York: Routledge

Winnicott D.W. (1950–55) 'Aggression in relation to emotional development' in *Through Paediatrics to Psychoanalysis*, London: Hogarth Press

Zetzel, E. (1953) 'The depressive position' in *The Capacity for Emotional Growth*, London: Maresfield Prints

Chapter 2

Destructiveness: revenge, dysfunction or constitutional evil?

Robert Royston

Introduction

What is the source of human destructiveness? Is it coded into our basic dynamism, a timbre in the child's first cry, natural, just as sucking for food is natural; or is it secondary, a reaction to stimulus? To put it slightly differently, is destructiveness a thing-in-itself, a primal energy, or is it generated by vulnerability, pain and unhappiness?

This question, upon which much rests, is perennial because it is incapable of resolution through appeals to logic or evidence. These two viewpoints, though not exclusive of each other, evoke two different images of the human species. To borrow from Heinz Kohut, the first depicts the human as guilty, predisposed to self-destructiveness, the second as tragic, vulnerable to damaging external forces.

But first, there are fundamental distinctions that must be made.

Destructiveness in psychoanalytic thinking is not the same as aggression.

Everyone is born with aggressive potential; diffuse aggression energises constructive actions. Eating has an aggressive component but is not destructive. The development of psychic boundaries relies on an aggressive distancing of self from other, but is constructive, psychologically healthy. Aggression mobilised against threat is protective of the subject and therefore constructive from the point of view of the attacked person.

Of course, aggression may also be destructive. Wars of conquest are damaging, but their aim is aggrandisement and, to the colonising power, they are glorious. The whole subject of destructiveness is intertwined around itself. Abusive violence is not consciously aimed at the self but at the other. However, the other is often a vessel into which the attacker projects a feared and hated part of the self. There is a common saying: when someone commits suicide the analyst asks, what other person was being murdered in the suicidal process; when someone kills, the question is, what part of themselves were they killing in the body of the other? In other words, murder, considered psychologically, is seldom simple. The other person is hated or despised or feared because they have come to represent a part of the attacker's personality. A hated part of the self, projected into the other, comes under murderous attack.

Aggression may target the subject directly, as in sado-masochism, or self-injury, or in various forms of self-sabotage. However, attacks on the self often have the transcendental goal of self-redemption. They are driven, perhaps, by guilt when their goal is purgation and relief. Sado-masochistic practices appear self destructive – the body is painfully and degradingly manipulated – but their aim is to alleviate mental pain and conflict through sexualised ritual. Perversions appear destructive to the aliveness of the natural self, but are sometimes defences against trauma, against a deflated and damaged self, against severe depression or disintegration, or are attempts to bind aggression, again through ritual and sexual feeling. They can be seen as attempted solutions.

However, there is another view entirely, which is that the assessment of the situation just given is blind to a secret force that invisibly enters the field of the perverse and takes it over. This is primary destructiveness. Primary destructiveness has not been neutralised by constructive drive energy and turned into healthy, useful aggression, instead it operates like a type of sinister agency in the life of the perverse patient and its hidden aim is to bring about empty deathlike states of mind.

This concept of destructiveness is controversial. Most therapists and analysts assert its non-existence, despite the foundational theories of Freud (1920) and Klein (1932, 1946), who from the start emphasised the pathogenic significance of aggression. What it is meant to be is a force whose motivation and aim is self-damage, the paralysis of the self, the retardation of psychic development, death in life or even physical death. An original impulse exists, which, if not harnessed by the ego, may gain powerful domination over psychic life and seek to kill development, liveliness, play, love, affection, contact with others and the sense of time. Like a torturer, it keeps the victim alive, merely so that it can continue its morbid existence, but, unlike a torturer, it anaesthetises the tortured subject. If the patient was cognisant of its malign effects, he or she would as it were wake up in dire alarm and combat the doleful self-annihilating enemy within.

Viewed in this way, destructiveness-for-its-own-sake comes to take on malevolent human shape and possess a cunning mind – it hides itself from its host, it generates defences, it seems to exist outside the control of the subject, in quite a different way to repressed unconscious content, by distorting the subject's sense of reality. It ceases to sound like a drive and becomes the psychological equivalent, if you like, of the devil.

Destructiveness for its own sake

Traditional views

The psychoanalytic argument in favour of destructiveness-for-its-own-sake does have a similar shape to ancient moral controversies and religious positions. It is a continuation of an old debate but with new evidence gained from clinical practice.

Traditional arguments place the location of evil either inside the psyche as a force, or outside as the impact of trauma. In the Garden of Eden story, evil arises from the destruction of primary innocence, which comes about as a result of disobedience and curiosity, weakness to temptation. The serpent or devil is external, but is invited into the human heart.

A slightly different Christian proposition is that people are born with an evil they must renounce along the path to moral regeneration, renouncing the Old Adam. This locates good, not evil, outside the person. After internal conflict, a wrestle with personal sin, we open the door of the heart to God, who subdues the hells within, and are regenerated.

Philosophical statements assert that man is born free, or is a noble savage, but everywhere in chains. Society, economics, the external state of things is a prisonhouse the newborn is delivered into. Here, too, evil, or destructiveness, begins outside the self. Evil is innocence traduced and damaged.

Destructiveness in psychological thinking

The abstract shape of these religious or philosophical views forms a substratum beneath psychoanalytical thinking. Destructiveness in psychoanalysis refers to a person's, a patient's, seemingly perverse tendency to reverse the logic of the pleasure principle and seek pain and cling to the past rather than change for the better. Borderline patients in particular are seen to resist the benign effects of insight and therapeutic care. These patients, it is said, forget, chop up, castrate, distort, crush and encapsulate insight: the more successful the therapy potentially is, the more destructive and immune to health the patient becomes, and seems to revel in this destruction of the therapeutic project and, more saliently, the therapist. In this process, envy of the therapist is said to be a feature and to be an aspect of the death instinct.

The argument is divided along inside/outside lines. Death instinct theory argues with what you might call real trauma theory; constitutional sadomasochism with the impinging environment. The death instinct view sees self-destruction as a disguised form of pleasure or at least as the expression of a pent-up basic instinct; the real trauma view sees it as arising from inflicted pain, an attempted solution to pain.

Each side may accuse the other of poor thinking. The real life viewpoint may deny psychic mechanism. A simplistic linear connection is made between pathogenic experience and psychopathology, ignoring each person's characteristic processes, what might be done with experience by people who function in different ways. One patient may react to deprivation by identifying with the abuser and, in covert ways, inflicting abuse on the self throughout later life; another may erect more self-protective defences.

The real trauma theorist would accuse opponents of tunnel vision, asserting they are so dazzled by the pathology of the patient's mental mechanisms, and their perversity, that they look no further, sweeping toxic childhood experience to the margins of the inquiry. It is, for example, possible to read detailed accounts of a patient's perverse internal reality in case studies that scarcely refer to childhood experience with caretakers. These might offer a sliver of history, which makes no contribution to the actual treatment, but nevertheless hints at fulsome pathogenic interaction between parent and child. From this particular analytic viewpoint pathological caretakers are considered of marginal importance. Attempts to focus on them, or relate the patient's difficulties to them, are seen as diversionary. It is what the patient does with the analyst's contribution that is the most, perhaps the only, important matter.

The debate is incapable of resolution. A robust response to these criticisms can be expected along these lines: 'We do not discount the impact of the environment even if the patient's mental mechanisms are the central focus. Constitutional self-destructiveness has to be bound and neutralised by the life instincts. The mother's nurturing presence is vital for this. If that fails then the death instinct, or whatever one might wish to call it, is unmodified and often takes the form of pathological and destructive narcissism.'

This line of thinking could go on to assert that there is a constituency of patients who have been abused and ill treated, but we all have a predisposition to destructiveness; there is a fascist part that wants to take over the good side of the self and dominate, with ruinous results. The cause of this setup lies in an archaic, mysterious infantile hinterland. The psyche is made up of selves in conflict and there may be a proliferation of evildoers acting within the larger whole-self. An example of a view along similar lines is offered by Hering (1997).

Conversely, it is said that death instinct theory blames the victim and in being blind to the adult perpetrator is by definition unempathic. The analyst, it is asserted, may be defending himself against the disturbing fact of abuse. Death instinct theory is not very different from Christian tirades against the devil. Criminals, for example, are not evil (though frightening and hateful) but themselves as much victims as the people they victimised. The internal world *is* made up of conflicting selves, some of which aim to persecute others, but this situation is the product of internalisations (Fairbairn 1943). The shadow of the object falls on the subject, as Freud (1917) said – self-destructiveness here is a distorted form of revenge. Often attacks on the self are attacks on objects subsumed into the self. An attack on the self replicates attacks made on the child by an abusive, neglectful or incompetent parent. The mind is history internalised and transformed into personality. (For an argument along somewhat similar lines, see DeZulueta 1997.)

And what, it may be lamented, about the sheer improbability of the death drive existing? Why even consider the possibility of such a drive?

Psychoanalytic theory and the death instinct

The first theoretical formulation in the direction of a death drive came in 1905 when Freud asserted the existence of a primal sado-masochistic impulse. Later in his clinical work he encountered stubborn and troubling forms of resistance and he felt the phenomena of the repetition compulsion threatened his magnificently detailed vision. The central feature of this vision was that the human mind and body sought pleasure, but had to adapt to a social environment and did so by repressing drives or trans-forming them into socially acceptable forms (sublimation). As things stood, psychoanalytic theory could not account for the difficulties that afflicted psychoanalytical therapy. The fact was that patients who should have been cured stayed where they were, as though they actually clung to pain rather than sought pleasure. More needed to be understood, thought Freud, and the product of his important reconsideration was the notion of the death instinct, formulated in 'Beyond the pleasure principle' (1920). His thoughts moved in the direction of a destructive component responsible for the anti-therapeutic conservatism of the mental apparatus of his patients, their tendency to cling to resistance, to the old, no matter how painful.

Psychoanalysis is concerned with the origin of mental states. Freud cast his mind back in his search for the most original of all sources of self-destruction, to prehistory, almost the prehistory of matter itself. He saw the death instinct, quintessentially, not as the teeming aggressiveness that characterised Klein's child patients and not as the powerful triumphant need to kill off the therapist's offerings, which we know so much about today, but as a cosmic nostalgia. He looked at the sexual drive. What was its goal? Relief. Yes, there is a massive heightening of pleasure, but the terminus of the sex urge is a state where there is no more sex urge. So he argued that all drives reached into the future with their cargo of desire and their intention was to abandon this load of painful tension and return, annihilated, to an earlier state of things: death, the state where no painful agitation itched inside the body. He divided libido into two poles. One was the life instinct, positive energy that seeks to unite things into larger and more creative wholes; the other was the death instinct, which seeks release from tension and the annulment of desire. The sexual instincts, which seek to preserve life, fight the death instinct by amalgamating with it and binding it and by turning it outwards in the form of aggression towards the other.

In a unique speculative passage, Freud conjures an image of a protozoic ocean of static life forms, where nothing changes, nothing disturbs timeless cosmic sleep, forms do not evolve, until the arrival of some type of external agent. The environment changes in some way and this creates a trigger.

Something in the atmosphere, say, mutates and, for the first time, the growth of living matter is a possibility. So the sleeping or original dead clay of matter stirs, the sleeping giant of life stirs, after its static prehistory and develops the potential to transmute into higher forms. Matter's sense of time begins. A perpetual and entirely null present tense now lives with two siblings, future and past. And this is the birth of the death instinct. Just as sexual desire cranes into the future and seeks to create new forms, so a cosmic nostalgia reaches backwards pulling things towards the inorganic, the original blissful quietude that preceded all growth and change.

An argument against this line of thinking would say that Freud's project in 'Beyond the pleasure principle' was impelled by clinical frustration and was far fetched. He attempted, as it were, to dismantle life energy, the psychic atom and in doing so postulated that a mysterious urge for the calm sleep of death lay at the core of this atom.

Objections proliferate. In the first place, Freud is attributing consciousness, memory and mind to dead matter. How can matter long for a former state of things when, being insentient, it could never have experienced that state of things. Raw matter was not ever conscious. It could never have enjoyed its own death sleep because it could never have been aware of it: conscious death is a contradiction in terms. A similar objection applies to Freud's idea when thought of in terms of drive rather than in terms of his metaphor about the planet and matter. How can the death instinct want to experience the death of its host organism when death is incapable of being conscious of itself? Freud, too, appears to attribute to mechanical energies something akin to a mind: memory, for example, and an ability to think and plan, plan the destruction of the life force. There seems to be a conflation here of libido, that is, raw energy, and human consciousness.

Yet the great struggle between the two forces of life and death takes place inside us without our awareness. In Freud's picture we come to look like hosts inside which busy entities and alien forces work silently. As described by Freud they come to seem increasingly like internal sub-selves or homunculi. The death instinct has a plan. This is to dismantle the life instinct in favour of regression to the big sleep. Life instinct has a plan, it is to defeat the death instinct, which it projects outwards, or binds – suddenly the many units of the psychobiological mind think complicated thoughts deep below our unconscious or preconscious mind.

Metapsychological drive theory itself points to a mysterious inner world of crypto-human energies as the source of mental disturbance and the type of destructiveness we have been talking about. Theory here begins to exclude people as causal factors, in favour of elemental conflict within drive itself. Here is a theory of pathology that excludes experience with damaging objects in favour of experience with damaging homunculi.

Initially, Freud was cautious. There was much in 'Beyond the pleasure principle' that was inspired guesswork to account for the strange facts of the repetition compulsion, negative therapeutic reaction and the tenacity of the transference. But, without intervening thought or dispute, the idea of constitutional destructiveness quite rapidly became an established part of theory, particularly in the work of Melanie Klein (1932) and others later, whose ideas were forged around the notion, not of real trauma entering from without, but of internal struggle with the constitutional serpent, the death instinct.

In an early phase, she said, the baby attacks the good that is the breast, in unconscious phantasy, burning, cutting splitting and mutilating it, soiling it with faeces. In a later phase, the baby, if it makes the right moral choice, offers reparation for its attacks on the external good. It enters the depressive position. The shattered images of the breast, the good thing, come together and the baby can be strengthened by this, rather than poisoned by the damage it itself has pushed into the breast. The attacks on the breast were driven by the death instinct. Whatever else happened along the developmental road there was this outpouring of constitutional death energy, as though from some nozzle or spark plug in the baby's energy grid.

In this idea the devil is within. Good, mother, is without. There is no sense of a malign outside world or any sign of stages and struggles later in childhood, unless those struggles are versions of the original conflict between internal evil and external good.

This idea had an effect on psychoanalytic theory and led to an impressive body of valuable ideas and case studies. But, in a way, how surprising it is that this should have happened. Surprising because of an absence of evidence conclusive enough to support such a profound assertion. Why *should* the infant's sadism be uncaused by external factors?

It might be argued that psychoanalytic drive theory in its original form inhibits our ability to understand the impact of the child's significant objects. Children internalise their caretakers, who become internal objects, or build up defensive systems to survive the pathogenic inroads of inadequate, hostile or abusive parents. Psychological distortions form in a struggle with outside people. Certain forms of drive theory have a tendency to divert attention from this fact onto the unhelpful things the patient does, without reference to external causes.

The concept of transference, for example, has changed. The transference, to Freud, was originally an acting out of amnesia. What was forgotten was repeated. Analysis of transference liberated memory. Transference is now more of an enclosed world in which there are only two protagonists, therapist and patient. The genetic interpretation that goes back to the past is often frowned on as a defensive displacement from the analyst onto substitute objects.

That said, the most extraordinary feature of Freud's cosmic vision in 'Beyond the pleasure principle' is its applicability in the consulting room. Matter yearns nostalgically for the inert mud bath of the inorganic. How true, the therapist may observe, who has been struggling for years with a patient's overwhelming desire for anti-therapeutic slumber. The death instinct idea in the consulting room has its most intense focus on the borderline patient's tenacious reinstatement of the old way. Therapeutic gains are made and then lost, dismantled. In this way the patient's efforts towards growth and development are ceaselessly undermined by negative therapeutic reaction. Analysis, interpretation itself, is attacked as if by a force that insists on a return to the past. Growth is ruthlessly cut down.

When this is challenged by interpretation a series of reactions may occur, which appear to vindicate the concept of the death instinct, or of aggression welling up from a profound source, and not caused by abuse or the environment in any direct way. The patient, for example, may dream of obscure processes in which a person about whom they have experienced a fleeting feeling of tenderness is reduced in a factory to inanimate matter and sealed in a lead pipe. It then may become evident that this is the fate, too, of all interpretations in so far as they are experienced as helpful, and particularly if they are thought to be achieved through empathy rather than intellect. Helpful comments are robbed of meaning. Emotional moments in the session are later doubted, minimised, distorted or forgotten. A deadly state of inanition is set up in the consulting room and no liveliness is possible.

The case

Someone opposed to the concept of the death instinct, contrariwise, might argue along these lines. A concern with destructiveness and perversity bypasses the patient's abusive objects. Of course, it may at times appear that the patient is implacably destructive of the object. The patient attacks *all* interpretations and the more helpful they are the more they are attacked. However, to attribute this to constitutional drives, to a visceral yearning for the mud bath of the inorganic, is to ignore the transference, a concept central to psychoanalytic practice. The destructive patient has climbed out of the role of the abused child into a zone of superiority. He feels he no longer needs anyone, but fears that if he abandons this self-sufficiency the therapist will change into the original abusive object and history will repeat itself.

The idea that the patient's attacks are fuelled by constitutional drive encourages the therapist to confront the patient's badness. But, the counter-argument might run, it also encourages an acting out of the transference on the analyst's part. The analyst instantly becomes the superego. The relationship between patient and therapist is inevitably distorted. Zealous tracking down of destructiveness involves an invasive transference dynamic that is rarely seen as transference, simply as robust analytical work. In fact, in the patient's experience the therapist is from the same mould as their attacking parent.

This contention might be rebutted in this way:

> You don't understand the nature of destructiveness that proceeds from the death instinct. The patient and I analyse experience with bad objects, external and internal, and effectively explore the transference. This works and there are gains, but the death instinct diagnosis comes into play because the patient destroys these gains. Again and again we find ourselves where we were before.
>
> We think about the death instinct when we think about the fate of interpretations. For example, a patient after disentangling herself from a highly disturbing relationship decided to phone the ex-boyfriend again to prove her freedom. The same destructive patterns were immediately triggered and the details of their interaction churned around in her head, keeping her awake at night. She started to drink heavily again and crashed her car. You can think as hard as you like about the patient's experiences with her father etc., but you will never explain why she brings it all back when it has been resolved, unless you invoke the idea of primary destructiveness, and particularly look at the deeply hidden payoff self destruction offers in terms of covert grandiosity. The death instinct mindset lords it over the humble human project of staying alive and trying to be happy. That's for suckers. The death instinct *is* the 'Übermensch'. It makes its own rules and despises the search for emotional growth.

And this destructiveness, this speaker would go on is always in tandem with fierce covert self-images. The woman I am talking about, for example, repeatedly dreamed of an executioner who revelled in decapitation. That was an image of her sultry power to destroy analytical thinking and castrate the therapist's ability to facilitate change. This is exactly along Freud's path: it is the working in the human psyche of matter's nostalgic pull backwards towards cosmic sleep before the arrival of the life instinct. You can call that poetical and melodramatic but it is a superbly accurate metaphor for what happens with some patients. Ignore that and you're letting everyone down.

Clinical example

The patient was a twice-divorced middle-aged man who had worked successfully in the City, and then extended his work into a network of investments abroad. He worked long and hard at this, but at the same time quickly became devoted to his sessions and struggled successfully to fit his work around them. He was in analytical therapy five times a week.

This man's core lifelessness was at first concealed behind a low-key manic façade, which often included a stream of light jokey patter, reference to television programmes and staccato laughter. As the therapy settled down, however, and after an initial period of constructive if superficial change, a deadening pattern emerged, characterised by accurate but unproductive analysis, insight not only without change but as a barrier to change. This was in the early days analysed as dissociation, intellectualisation, as an avoidance of the therapeutic encounter in favour of a scenario where two colleagues discuss an absent person, who to all intents and purposes might not even exist. These analyses, too, naturally, were subsumed into the patient's modus vivendi, which was stoically passive and monotonous and persistent. It was analysed fruitlessly as envy of the therapist's liveliness and potential productivity.

At first appearance this was a schizoid state, leeched of emotion, described by Guntrip (1968) as a withdrawal from emotional interaction and dependency due to the failure of the patient's objects. This diagnosis was consolidated by the patient's meek acceptance of my suggestions, and his malleability and quietness. However, it became obvious that he was effortlessly vitiating the analysis, most obviously by forgetting or changing his mind about important therapeutic experiences, returning next day with a radically different take on matters.

To this patient, I was fragile, frightened and sad, but noble in my conscientiousness (never late), stoical (never ill). However, to him, I struggled bravely to understand things and had to be preserved and protected in a hushed zone from which all light and conflict were excluded. A pall descended. A null pattern was established, occasionally broken by periods of empty jokiness. Language and even analysis itself, mutated into another identity. Words were used to eviscerate emotion or as a deadening interpersonal barrier. Speech took on a funereal quality and warded off conflict and emotion. Truth was not excluded, but its function mutated. The patient, in a sense, hid behind insight. The more the insight, the less the change.

This gives a negative impression of the patient, but, in fact, he was admirable in many ways and entirely innocent. The processes described appeared to happen to him. When we focused on them he would describe them with endless insight, but they continued to constitute a series of psychological mini-events and it was remarkable to witness the peculiar way in which the destructive dynamic appeared to have a life of its own, but in addition operated in this way because of the patient's attitude to it, which was secretly accommodating. The mechanism of disavowal was in operation, so the patient appeared passive but in another way was complicit, but blindly so.

It was sometimes a struggle to resist the mood this generated of contentless serenity. It was as though he and I constituted a hushed and silky continuum. We were pleasantly and seamlessly fused. I sometimes felt hypnotised, lulled and easeful and that his urgent problems were miles away.

What personal problems did this patient present? He said he felt he was living someone else's life, that he'd borrowed a job and a body. He felt vaguely but persistently doomed and anxious, but through a veil that was like a zone of sleep or happy easefulness. A quiet horror occasionally seized him that he lived outside time and the life process. He felt old, he said, but without experience. A repetitive dream revolved around the theme that he had been alive in previous ages and had experienced much, but was now a ghost with no memory. This sense of exoneration from ordinary time conferred a mood of superiority, as well as of loftiness over the grubby masses who toiled and aged and hungered and suffered and made plans for the future.

Clearly, in terms of the argument in this chapter, several questions emerge at once.

- The threat and sense of doom – is it a fear of the death instinct itself, an awareness of self-destruction or of an abusive childhood object?
- His sense of superiority, is it a culture of the death instinct that is itself invisible but observable by its products (Rosenfeld 1988) or a defensive superstructure shielding a narcissistically depleted or emotionally abused self; and was it that he and I had to be seamlessly fused so that I didn't turn into the object that destroyed the self?
- The contentless serenity of the sessions – is this a product of the death instinct, which has hollowed out the therapy, destroyed it as creative and locked him and I into a psychologically elite zone (only fools have conflictful analysis directed towards a better future, and hunger and struggle, but he and I are perfect), or is it there to exclude a predator, who is, as a result, miles away?

It is at precisely this point that the argument about the death instinct swallows itself. The patient's childhood was dominated by autocratic and single-minded caretakers who lacked empathy and sympathy and believed that the parent generation had a duty to hand down its experience and ideas to the next. This was done with cold, dead persistence. Neither parent made allowances for the struggles of the child and the learning process. Physical punishments were administered until a late age and were triggered by behaviour that asserted the child's developing self and independence and opinions. So, of course the patient was dominated by a persecuting object. Needless to say, shame and humiliation, rather than pride and satisfaction, attended growth and development and change. And, quite obviously, the patient's parents considered themselves and their opinions superior and timeless and invulnerable to change of any sort, and this was not only introjected by the patient, but pushed into him from without.

All of which powerfully answers the question in favour of the conclusion that the destructiveness existed in its original form outside the patient, like the chains that await Jean Jacques Rousseau's child who is born free. The environment is the first cause. Obviously, the child isn't a blank cheque and has individual processes and, clearly, another child might have dealt with the destructive stimuli differently, but surely would not have fared a lot better.

Of course, the patient projected into me his fragile self and made me experience what he had experienced – the scything down of growth processes. What happened was that the patient identified with the aggressor and possibly heightened the attack as a form of mute protest which, if it could speak, would say: look, this is what you've done to me. Here was protest and revenge operating in the form of self-destructiveness.

This conclusion needs to be thrown into the cage of its opponent, however, because there is much more to say. An opponent of the view above might argue as follows.

> Why didn't the therapy work more quickly and simply? Life is short and analysis long, but change does take place within a timeframe. Protracted analysis means the death instinct is in play. Everything you say is right, but what occurred was the dismantling of progress. You analysed this in terms of his relationship with you as the transference object and dealt with his sense that you invaded him with your interpretations; you worked with the idea that he had to push you out in order to preserve the self, but this exploration too fell victim to the malaise. The fact is, there was in the mix a ghostly, deadly entity that functioned like Freud's death instinct. This entity wasn't a revenge motive, it wasn't a defence. The patient worked tirelessly to prevent its identification. This third force has to be persistently taken up.

There is some truth in this idea. When the destructive processes were brought into sharp focus a spectrum of resistances came into play. These were dedicated to preserving the destructiveness and the narcissistic systems and ideas that accompanied it.

Such resistances take common forms:

- The patient redistributes causality, blaming the destructive processes on genetics (I was made that way), on psychoanalysis itself (the way it is set up prevents spontaneity and growth) or bypasses the fact of the self-damaging behaviour by immediately saying, 'yes, but why do I do it, that's what I want to know?' This last defence blames a cause that, because it is mysterious, cannot be to do with the patient in any salient way; he is a puppet of the cause.
- The patient may take up the position of the victim. He or she may become upset and weep in a way meant to establish the therapist or psychoanalysis as the abuser and the patient an abused innocent.

Sometimes, this type of weeping is meant to assert that the patient is a victim of his own nature. However, the weeping has no emotional depth.

- The patient changes the subject and introduces another more superficial problem and works on it plausibly, in a manner that emphasises constructive engagement.
- The patient works constructively with the problem but the next session the insights have been distorted or forgotten. This process is often accompanied by dramatic dreams. In one such dream, a man ate ravenously, but the more he ate the thinner he became. Then followed a scene with a man on a toilet who exploded with rage and the walls were covered with excrement and the man put on weight. In the dream of another patient, a highly impressive machine uprooted forests. In yet another dream, a man sat in a chair and listened to another man whom he could not see. The listening man became soft and pulpy. His facial features melted and at the end of this process he was a tube containing pulped flesh and crushed bones.

I think these images show that the mental mechanisms lined up against the content of the analysis are powerful and mentally violent. There is an element of omnipotence. The patient has an invulnerable ability to reorder reality in the mind, to reverse the roles of aggressor and attacked, to generate a plausible culture that supports the innocence of the self, to subjectively change the objective world into an acceptable form. The patient, in other words, is not a slave to the truth. He may well be skilled at pulling others into collusion with the culture of self-exoneration. So, while the patient may be a genuinely excellent citizen, and in many ways admirable, his psychodynamic processes come to resemble those commonly detected in offenders and people who do abuse others.

What this shows, to the clinician who believes destructiveness is *sui generis*, is that the death instinct has a sinister intelligence that works to protect itself from any sort of challenge that might lead to its dissolution. Two reality factors threaten the death instinct. One is recognition of the personal damage it causes; the other is guilt, or the recognition of damage to the other. Tireless work is often put in by the patient to avoid recognising these realities.

Does that mean that the argument must resolve on the side of the death instinct? A clinical phenomenon stands in the way of this conclusion, which is that if the therapy ends successfully, it has always been the case, in my experience, that destructiveness, in retrospect, appears defensive. When it pales, another stratum of experience and the mind emerges. This is the subself that was hiding behind the narcissistic death instinct-driven self. This self needs to rely on the analysis in a new way and be looked after and fed, de-traumatised, if it can be put like that.

What is thought of as the death instinct is part of a narcissistic system. This has a flourishing secret life of its own and is peopled by an unconscious spectrum of grandiose and often violent self-images. The system does not at first appear defensive, but does so later, when the vulnerable underlying self is allowed to come to the surface. The narcissistic system was defensive but offered the patient a compensatory sense of power, triumph and excitement. These last factors made the system particularly tenacious.

The theoretical argument does not end there. A counterargument states that constitutional destructiveness uses what is there. It is only after the analysis of the death instinct that one enjoys the luxury of discounting its existence.

Conclusion

In conclusion, my own view on the death instinct is that, in the field of theory, the notion should be rejected, but with profound caution; in clinical practice, it should be treated with suspicion and definitely allowed a place, but as a metaphor. The death instinct is a necessary fiction.

Even if there is constitutional destructiveness, another level exists. Here destructiveness operates powerfully and its origin is interpersonal. Whatever the patient might add, the original impetus towards self-damaging behaviour comes from toxic experiences with caretakers. The patient may attack the therapist out of envy. However, the most potent source of envy is the narcissistic adult who demands admiration. Revenge may be a factor and the patient's body, mind and life may symbolise the abusive or negligent childhood object and may be attacked accordingly.

References

DeZulueta, F. (1997) 'Demonology versus science', *British Journal of Psychotherapy* 14(2): 199–205

Fairbairn, W.R.D. (1943) *Psychoanalytic Studies of the Personality*, London: Routledge & Kegan Paul

Freud, S. (1917) 'Mourning and melancholia', *Standard Edition 14*, London, Hogarth Press

—— (1920) 'Beyond the pleasure principle', *Standard Edition 13*, London: Hogarth Press

—— (1905) 'Three essays on the theory of sexuality', *Standard Edition 7*, London: Hogarth Press

Guntrip, H. (1968) *Schizoid Phenomena, Object Relations and the Self*, London: Hogarth Press

Hering, C. (1997) 'Beyond understanding? Some thoughts on the meaning and function of the notion of "evil"', *British Journal of Psychotherapy* 14(2): 209–220

Klein, M. (1932) *The Psycho-Analysis of Children*, London: Hogarth Press

—— (1946) 'Notes on some schizoid mechanisms' in *Envy and Gratitude and other Works 1946–1963*, London: Hogarth Press and the Institute of Psychoanalysis

Rosenfeld, H. (1988) 'A clinical approach to the psychoanalytic theory of the life and death instincts: an investigation into the aggressive aspects of narcissism' in *Melanie Klein Today, Volume 1*, E. Bott Spillius (ed.), London and New York: Routledge

Part II

Developmental and theoretical perspectives

Chapter 3

From biting teeth to biting wit: the normative development of aggression[1]

Marianne Parsons

> [A] little girl of three, in the throes of a struggle with her rather wild aggressive nature . . . returned one day from nursery school to report triumphantly on her 'good' behaviour in the group: 'Not hit, not kick, not bit, only spit!'
>
> (Freud, A. 1972: 163)

The concept of aggression is one of the most controversial in psychoanalytic theory. Views range from seeing aggression as an instinctual drive on a par with libido, the derivation of the death instinct, an expression of the self-preservative instincts, a reaction to environmental influences. It can be understood in terms of activity, adaptation and mastery, and as destructive and pathological. The theoretical viewpoint we take profoundly affects our clinical understanding and technique.

The capacity for aggression is essential for psychic growth. The healthy development of the self and the capacity to separate and individuate require aggressive activity. Like sexuality, aggression can be used constructively and progressively or destructively and regressively. Its appropriateness in any specific situation depends on the manner of its expression and the developmental level of the individual. For example, it is age appropriate for a toddler to have tantrums, but not the older child or adolescent. In situations of real danger, violent aggression to protect the self or others may be entirely appropriate. By the same token, such behaviours as unprovoked violence, sadism, contemptuous denigration, bullying and wanton destructiveness are largely regressive and arise from pathology not health. Because of their regressive and pathological nature there is no developmental line for such destructive behaviours. By contrast, one can conceive of a developmental line of normative healthy aggression and an attempt will be made in

---

1 This chapter to be published in 2006 in *Clinical Lectures in Delinquency, Perversion and Violence*, S. Ruszczynski and D. Morgan (eds), London: Karnac.

this chapter to trace this, together with some of the influences that can throw it off course.

Winnicott's view was that aggression arises from environmental impingements, especially traumatic early object experiences, as well as instinctual forces (Winnicott 1950–55). Summarising a panel on aggression, Heimann and Valenstein wrote:

> Our psychoanalytic experience tells us that certain patients who show particular problems with aggression have had to suppress or otherwise defend themselves in infancy and childhood from environmental influences that were not conducive to the progression of their developmental needs for the normal expression of aggression.
>
> (1972: 34)

The power of love to bind hatred is crucial. People showing pathological aggression tend to be those who were not enabled in childhood to develop a secure libidinal attachment in which they felt loved and contained by primary caretakers. Institutionalised children with multiple caretakers, traumatised children and those who have suffered severe physical pain, neglect or over-stimulation and children for whom fear has been a daily currency may show the kind of uncontrollable, apparently senseless destructiveness otherwise only seen in brain-damaged and psychotic children. Anna Freud noted that the pathological factor in such cases was not the aggressive tendencies themselves, but a lack of fusion between the aggressive and libidinal urges:

> The pathological factor is found in the realm of erotic, emotional development which has been held up through adverse external or internal conditions, such as absence of love objects, lack of emotional response from the adult environment, breaking of emotional ties as soon as they are formed, deficiency of emotional development for innate reasons. Owing to the defects on the emotional side, the aggressive urges are not brought into fusion and thereby bound and partially neutralised, but remain free and seek expression in life in the form of pure, unadulterated, independent destructiveness . . . The appropriate therapy has to be directed to the neglected, defective side, i.e. the emotional libidinal development.
>
> (1949: 41–2)

There is a danger of equating adult behaviours, feelings and phantasies with those of children. Something may look actively destructive to our adult eye, but we should not assume that destructive intent (as we know it) is necessarily in the young child's mind. The child's capacity for mental functioning is limited at every developmental stage by his awareness of himself and his knowledge of the world around him. Does the tiny baby who screams and kicks have destructive intent or is he in some primitive bodily way trying to get rid of intolerable feelings? Edgcumbe (1976) addressed this question succinctly:

> The baby's wish to get rid of nasty experiences may be viewed as the earliest form of mental aggressiveness in the sense that it involves a primitive hostile reaction to something unpleasant. The very young baby, however, cannot tell what the something is, where it comes from, or what, if wishing does not work, will make it go away. He cannot distinguish between feelings arising in his own body and stimuli coming from outside.
>
> (1976: vii)

The baby gradually begins to differentiate 'me' from 'not-me' and inner experience from external stimuli, learning over time that his cries prompt his mother to do something to relieve his distress. When his cries go unheard and his needs unmet, he begins to feel frustrated. The baby needs 'perfect adaptation at the theoretical start, and then needs a carefully graduated failure of adaptation' (Winnicott 1950–55: 216). Crucial for the development of the sense of a real self and the capacity for healthy relationships are the opposition mother offers to the young child, the importance of the child's experience of aggression and the need for fusion between erotic love and aggression (Winnicott 1950–55). Aggression therefore operates both in the service of self-preservation and survival *and* development.

The development of aggression is closely connected with many aspects of the child's development: psychosexual, object relations, ego and superego, cognitive capacities and the integration of his sense of self. All these contribute to the child's abilities (or not) to tolerate, process and deal with his aggressive feelings at every stage of development. There are developmentally appropriate phantasies and means of expressing, defending against and dealing with aggression – hence the title of this chapter, which implies a movement from bodily to symbolic expression.

Infancy – 'from biting teeth . . .'

In the oral phase of infancy, feeling hungry, feeling full, swallowing, biting, spitting, vomiting, gurgling, cooing and crying play a key role in the experience and expression of pleasure and unpleasure (Freud 1920). Privation or frustration of basic needs and of a sense of going-on-being (Winnicott 1963a) can arouse primitive anxieties of disintegration and annihilation. Observation indicates that the earliest forms of aggression are triggered by such primitive *anxieties*, not by wilful innate destructiveness.

The adult's loving expression 'I could eat you!' aptly mirrors the aggressive possessive love that the baby has for his mother (stemming originally, we imagine, from his attitude towards her feeding breast). This aggressive possessive love can be seen in the way children love their most beloved toys 'to death', biting off their ears, flinging them aside, then retrieving and clutching them passionately. At this stage of development, it is *aggressive love* not *hatred* that threatens destruction (Freud, A. 1949). The baby's intimacy with the mother is conducted primarily through bodily expressions. Typical signs of protest are gaze avoidance, refusing food and squirming when being held. Self-directed aggression (biting, head banging and hair pulling) is unusual and indicates disturbance (Hoffer 1949):

> From this stage of development onwards it is essential for the child's normality that the aggressive urges should be directed away from the child's own body to the animate or inanimate objects in the environment . . . At a later stage aggression will normally be used again in a self-destructive manner. But it will then be invested in the superego and directed against the ego itself, not against the body.
>
> (Freud, A. 1949: 40)

Although babies may be endowed with differing strengths of aggressive drive, the impact of the environment on the child's capacity to deal with aggressive forces is crucial. How babies begin to make sense of their feelings and experiences depends largely on the way mother perceives and relates to them, which will be affected by her own internal world and experiences of self and other. The mother's capacity to empathise with and help her baby manage his greedy demands will be impaired if she feels too plagued by his cries, experiencing them as attacks. This will impede the baby's healthy aggressive development:

> When a tiny baby feels hungry or frightened he has no resources for making himself feel better and has to rely on his caregivers. If his needs are not adequately met, his distress, helplessness and sense of frustration will become overwhelming. He will yell and cry, kick and flail his arms. This constitutes the earliest mode of response to an overwhelming experience, namely a bodily one. The crucial thing from the point of view of development is the nature of the mother's response. Good-enough mothering will give the baby sufficiently often an experience of not yelling and flailing into a vacuum, but of having elicited a response that alleviates his distress. This is more than the meeting of a need; it is the meeting up with an empathic and receptive object. It lays the foundations for the capacity to tolerate vulnerability because helplessness is associated with a protective object.
>
> (Parsons & Dermen 1999: 330–31)

The good-enough mother acts as a protective shield (Freud 1920; Khan 1973) by empathic attunement to her baby and by trying to relieve her baby's pain and anxiety until he gradually develops the resources to do this for himself. This enables the baby to develop a sense of basic safety and trust, to have pleasurable experiences with the mother and to form a secure attachment to her. Not only does the baby feel loved, but also develops over time a capacity to attune to his own internal states, tolerate his needs and differentiate between shades of feeling until not every internal state has the same urgency. Prolonged absence of the mother's protective function exposes the baby to unmanageable amounts of anxiety that can lead to a deviant course of aggression and patterns of relating (Fraiberg 1982). A mother's protective function may be inadequate for many reasons, for example, depression, unresolved conflicts over her own aggression, unconscious hostility to her baby, lack of support from her partner.

As the baby begins to develop a sense of self-agency (Stern 1985), the good-enough mother intuitively recognises that her baby can tolerate more frustration and can exercise his curiosity and do more things for himself. She continues to 'feel with' her baby (Furman 1992) but, instead of immediately managing her baby's feelings for him, she gives him more space to begin to learn how to manage his own feelings and experiences. The baby begins to internalise her protective function. Repeated experiences of optimal frustration in the context of empathic mothering help him learn that he can survive feelings of helplessness without being overwhelmed. This promotes the development of healthy aggression.

A vignette from mother–infant observation illustrates a baby's aggressive reaction to anxiety, fear and distress within a good-enough mother–child relationship:

> K is 10 months old. Her mother went away for three days and she slept a lot during this time. When the mother returned K did not look at her, only at the window, and when the mother went to the car to collect her luggage, K cried and cried in absolute despair as if it was all too much for her to bear. For the next three days K guarded the door, but then was able to settle and feel safe again. When I visited one week later, K came to greet me with her shoe in her hand. We had played a very nice game with her shoe on previous visits – she would give it to me and I would give it back. At first I thought she wanted to play the game again, but this time she came closer to me, holding the shoe in the air. I thought she was going to hit me so I made a move to defend myself, but she just stopped in front of me holding the shoe high in the air. She looked at me seriously, then turned round, crawled over to the wall and began to hit the wall with the shoe. Her mother said, 'No, K, that will mark the wall.' K listened to her and stopped hitting the wall, then went over to her toys. She began to throw her toys in the air, listening

to the hard noise they made as they fell to the floor. The mother seemed to understand K's state of mind and said, 'Good girl!'

(Pohjamo, personal communication, 1994)

K's aggressiveness seems to stem from her reaction to mother's absence. Although not physically aggressive towards her mother, she had clearly been distressed (she could not look at mother when she returned, cried in absolute despair, then guarded the door for three days). When the observer arrives – someone who regularly comes and goes – we can imagine K remembering her feelings about mother's absence and return and surmise that K's aggression towards mother is displaced in her aggressive approach to the observer. But instead of attacking she displaces her aggression onto the wall. When mother prohibits this, she displaces her aggressive feelings further into a game, throwing her toys and enjoying the hard noise they make. The observer senses that mother knows that K is displacing her aggressive feelings onto inanimate objects as she encourages this adaptive behaviour by praising her for being a 'good girl'. Perhaps K's secure relationship with her mother enables her to remember her love for mother and wish to please her even in the face of aggressive feelings towards her, i.e. the foundations of the fusion between libidinal and aggressive urges.

Toddlers

The toddler continues to express aggression via the body (biting, kicking, pinching, throwing things) and through screams and yells because he has not yet developed the mental resources for processing and managing feelings of frustration and anger. Prior to developing the capacity for concern for the object, the toddler revels in a sense of powerful agency and some cruelty is to be expected at this age (Winnicott 1963b). Cruelty to animals is not uncommon: the family pet often needs to be rescued both from the toddler's attacks and his aggressive love. Toddlers feel omnipotent, resent being controlled or having to share. They delight in being messy, noisy, powerful and aggressive. Aggression is triggered especially by assaults on the child's omnipotence, by fear of loss of the object and of the object's love and by core complex anxieties of feeling abandoned or engulfed (Glasser 1996). Advances in ego development allow for a wider variety of defences. For example, when the toddler's messy or cruel wishes conflict with their internal and/or external world, he may deal with them by attempting to transform them into the opposite through 'reaction formation'. Thus cruelty may be transformed into pity, kindness and protectiveness. Reaction formation is a very adaptive, civilising defence; but if overused or used precociously, it can lead to maladaptive ways of defending against aggressive impulses such as pathological self-sacrifice, perfectionism and obsessionality.

At this stage, magical thinking holds sway: to wish something makes it happen. There is no clear distinction between reality and phantasy or between internal and external events. So, the angry toddler who is left by mother may imagine that his wish to get rid of her made her disappear. It takes time to sort this out. It also takes time for the toddler to learn that the adults perceive some things they do while exploring their environment as dangerous, destructive or naughty. The toddler faces the confusing problem:

> [W]hich of his many activities are really destructive or aggressive, and which are potentially useful and creative? In normal development the child gradually arrives at some kind of working definition that allows him to distinguish between those of his actions which are actually harmful and those which are not.
>
> (Edgcumbe 1976: x)

During healthy toddlerhood the child begins to assert more independence by actively doing more for himself, in *his* way. But the toddler also wants to please mother because his well-being depends on her love. He faces a major conflict of ambivalence as he experiences violent swings between love and hate. He hates mum when she does not gratify him but loves her when she comforts and provides for his needs. When the toddler feels hatred, his sense of loving and being loved may disappear. Such intense feelings arise in relation to many age-appropriate developmental conflicts. Toilet training is an obvious example where faeces (a loving gift or a noxious weapon) may be used as an expression of love or aggression in the mother–child relationship. (Derivatives of this type of anal aggressiveness sometimes persist into later life as expressions of contempt. In extreme forms they appear in some types of criminality, e.g. the burglar who literally leaves shit everywhere.) If the mother can manage her toddler's anger and hatred without feeling narcissistically wounded, without retaliating and without needing to deny his negative feelings towards her, she offers him a model for dealing with ambivalence. Through internalisation of her capacities, the child integrates his loving views of the mother with the angry and hostile ones and recognises that the mum who is sometimes angry with him also still loves him. This integration of loving and hating feelings is crucial for the healthy development of aggression. It enables the child to develop a sense of trust that his affectionate relationship with mother will endure during moments of anger and separations from her. Without such integration, 'omnipotent and magical ways of thinking will persist unmodified, the power of love to tame destructiveness will be diminished, and the child's belief in the enormity of his aggression will be unchecked' (Parsons & Dermen 1999: 333).

Increasingly, the mother has to say 'no' to stop the toddler in order to protect him from danger, or to protect herself and others from his aggressive behaviour. He *must not* bite his sister or make a mess, he *should* use the potty, put on his coat etc. Such limits and demands make him feel frustrated and angry forcing him to recognise that he is not all powerful and will not be gratified unconditionally. This painful blow to his previously omnipotent sense of himself arouses enormous frustration and often results in the temper tantrums typical in toddlerhood. The toddler in a tantrum can feel overwhelmed and out of control and needs the continuous presence of the adult to help him regain composure. Being angrily controlled or left alone in such a state leaves the child at the mercy of unmanageable panic and does not help him to learn ways of containing and dealing with his frustration and aggression. The parents' ability to treat the child with respect and enable him to feel a 'somebody' (Furman 1992) while imposing restraints offers the child a model for internalisation, whereby he can develop an active sense of self and self-respect and an acceptance of limits.

Observations from a mother–toddler group illustrate the development of aggression at this stage. Mrs A, a loving and attentive mother, was anxious to avoid any confrontation with Tom. Nervous of any signs of aggression, she was never firm with him, but she was very controlling in her attempts to help him. Tom was very tied to her and wanted to be babied. He could not assert himself and found no delight in age-appropriate aggressive play or behaviour.

> Just before he was 2, Tom made a tower of blocks. His mother intervened to show him how to place them correctly. He built as directed, then pushed over the tower without any delight. Very cautiously he began to build again, but doing it his way with the blocks in a haphazard fashion.
>
> Two weeks later, Tom had found a little more self-assertiveness. Tom put the little Russian dolls together in the wrong order, and his mum repeatedly showed him the correct way, explaining carefully all the time. Finally, Tom covered the doll's face with another piece and shouted triumphantly, 'Can't talk!'

Good for Tom! His first moves towards self-assertion and individuation were a struggle, but gradually he became more independent and assertive. His fantasy play provided an imaginative outlet for the expression of his aggressive urges, his need to feel in control and his burgeoning thoughts about being a phallic boy. When Tom's father began to spend more time with him, their deeper relationship facilitated Tom's capacity to individuate from the intense and rather intrusive relationship with mother. He began to develop a stronger masculine identification and his fantasy play took on a more aggressive and phallic quality, with age-appropriate games and stories about guns and swords.

The parents' capacity to tolerate and manage their own frustration and aggression allows them to perceive their child's aggression as that of a child and enables them to respond appropriately as an adult instead of reacting on the basis of their own childlike needs and impulses. They offer experiences of forgiveness and reparation that promote the development of a healthy and non-punitive superego and the way in which they defend against their own aggression will be internalised by the child. The child has repeated opportunities to see that aggression may be felt but not acted on, expressed in an assertive but not damaging way or channelled into other activities. He learns that language is usually more appropriate than bodily expressions of aggression. All this promotes the child's natural urge to master feelings, conflicts and anxieties which, in turn, enhances his self-esteem and sense of well-being.

The nursery school child

At this age the child is particularly preoccupied with curiosity about sexual differences and wishes to be big, strong and admired. In boys this centres especially on physical and phallic power, in girls it is more about power to possess and exclude others. Aggression may be triggered by anxiety over loss of love, jealousy, envy and castration anxiety, and especially by affronts to the child's narcissism (causing him to feel shamefully small, humiliated and like a dependent baby). Interestingly, the majority of violent adult men seen at the Portman Clinic in London have severe problems with phallic narcissism.

Strides in ego development offer an increasing array of defences for dealing with unwelcome wishes, impulses and fantasies. One of the most common is externalisation, which 'gives the problem' to someone or something else – the childhood version of 'not me, guv!' – whereby the child can feel virtuous by identifying someone else as the naughty, aggressive or guilty one. However, the problem can easily ricochet back onto the child when externalisation extends to projection: the child then fears attack from the one he imbued with aggression. This is the source of many typical childhood fears of ghosts, monsters, wild animals and burglars. If defences for dealing with aggressive urges break down and aggressive wishes threaten to become conscious, nightmares may ensue and anything that might trigger conflictual feelings (such as stories, TV programmes, fantasy play, competitive and physical games) may become a source of fear to be avoided. The child may become phobic and inhibited. Aggression may be turned against the self and the child may become accident prone.

Some aggression is essential for separation. If the child's ego cannot tolerate aggressive feelings because they seem too dangerous, he may be unable to separate. For example, the child may fear leaving mum to start school because of his unconscious death wishes towards her, so he has to stay by her side to ensure that she remains safe. This is at the root of much school refusal and school phobia in childhood and adolescence.

I have been referring to defences that may be adaptive in the service of development or maladaptive impeding development. What of children without defences against aggression? At the mercy of their impulses, all hell will break loose: not only do they damage people and things, they also damage relationships and the chance of having experiences that help them to feel good about themselves. Material about Charles illustrates this:

> Charles, aged 6, was referred for analysis because of eruptive aggression, an inability to relate to peers and alarming swings between infantile behaviour and pseudo-mature language. He was terrified of abandonment, perceiving himself as a 'devil' hated by his parents. He was sure I would hate him too. His physical attacks on me were very violent: sometimes he behaved like a wild animal, spitting, biting, kicking, hurling toys, smearing faeces. His apparently unprovoked and unpredictable attacks were not simply manifestations of rage, but enactments of his internal chaos driven by *panic*. In time I understood that he was experiencing *me*, in the transference, as the source of danger. He enacted his internal chaos because he lacked resources for processing his emotional experiences in symbolic form, either through play or words, and he had no effective defences in the face of overwhelming internal states. Interpretation only heightened his anxiety and hence his aggression, instead of offering relief. By surviving without retaliating, by trying to offer a sense of safety and containment and by trying to let him know that I wanted to help not harm him, it gradually became possible to find a therapy 'language' that made words meaningful yet safe. When he was relatively calm and not actually 'spilling' out his chaos, I tried to empathise with his need for 'body talk' to express his 'spilly feelings'. My aim was both to keep him safe and enable him to begin to internalise a protective function. The first step was to help him to recognise an impending danger (approach of 'spilly feelings'), which would allow him to prepare himself by using anxiety as a signal (Freud 1926). The next step was to help him find some appropriate defences to deal with his anxiety. Gradually he began to express and explore his terrifying phantasies in play rather than violent 'body talk'. The gradual development of signal anxiety, together with his emerging capacities for some symbolic play, for differentiating reality from fantasy and for using words meaningfully, provided him with resources for developing appropriate defences to deal with his anxiety and aggression.

Charles was a very disturbed child who seemed to have had the worst of both worlds: an intensely powerful aggressive drive coupled with an uncontaining and often hostile environment. He felt hated by his parents and his mother's unconscious death wishes towards him were palpable. His emotional development was severely delayed and lacking the phallic-narcissistic and oedipal characteristics typical for a child of his age (Edgcumbe & Burgner 1975).

Normally, nursery school-aged children are passionately curious about their own and others' genitals and they puzzle about their functions. The mental images aroused by this confusion may lead them to imagine sexual activity as fighting. The child's longings for admiration, together with his passionate and aggressive interest in sexual activity, come to a head at the oedipal level in a conflict between his active wish to possess one parent exclusively and his anxiety about damaging his rival, the other parent. He wants to get rid of the rival, but fears retaliation for his aggressive wishes. He also faces the thorny problem that his rival is someone he still loves and needs. In a good-enough family environment, children find some resolutions of this dilemma by using their increasing capacities for rational thinking, reality testing, frustration tolerance and delayed gratification. Further ego development promotes capacities for symbolisation and distinguishing between reality and fantasy, allowing aggressive urges to be channelled through fantasy and play.

Physical expressions of aggression are still common at this stage, but the healthy child will increasingly use language to hurl insults. Repetitive chanting such as 'Silly you! Silly poo!' is typical. Although some cruelty to animals is expectable in toddlerhood, such cruelty in the nursery-aged child is usually a sign that the fusion of aggression with love and concern has stalled, causing the normative development of aggression to veer off course.

Latency

Physical aggression tends to be more purposeful and within fairly well-defined limits, unlike the rather random quality typical in younger children. Playground fights involving both physical and verbal aggression are quite commonplace in latency. If cruelty to animals persists into latency, serious disturbance is indicated. Persistent physical aggression is now a cause for concern.

In early latency, when the superego is not yet fully internalised, children believe firmly that others should be fair to them, but that they need not be fair to others. Aggression in competitive games takes the form of guiltless cheating, until the superego becomes more consolidated and the importance of fairness all round takes root. The child begins to adhere to the unwritten code that it is wrong to attack someone smaller or weaker; to take what is not yours and one against many is unfair. Children without the kind of internal world and good-enough home environment that promotes this kind of fair-minded thinking and capacity to restrain aggressive impulses, may show signs of delinquency and unrestrained aggression and may become bullies.

With some resolution of oedipal conflicts and solid foundations for gender identity, the development of the healthy latency child moves apace. His sense of self as capable of *doing* things and *being* someone progresses alongside the development of the ego ideal. Progressive ego and superego capacities provide the child with a broader variety of defences and offer more adaptive means of mastering and channelling his impulses and processing feelings. Language plays a central role in the expression of aggression and the child channels his energies into fantasy, constructive play and learning. Competitiveness is directed into sports and typical latency activities, such as collecting things. The passionate hunger for information and activities reveals the sublimation of instinctual urges. Developing the capacity for sublimation is a remarkable achievement and opens up new horizons for self-enhancing interests and activities, often giving pleasure not only to the child but others too. However, development does not proceed this smoothly for some children whose progress is impeded by their defences:

Ben, aged 7, was referred for treatment because his parents were worried about his wish to dress up as a girl in fantasy games. He was anxious about separating from his mum, jealous of his older sister and his little brother and, although usually very quiet, he would sometimes explode in rage. His wish to act the baby at home irritated his mother enormously. For many weeks in therapy he arranged the toy cars or animals in a long line, then moved the first car forward an inch followed by each car next in line. He then repeated the whole painstaking process again and again. It was painful and deadly boring to watch and terribly sad to see his tremendous anxiety about his sexual and aggressive impulses reflected in his inhibited and strictly controlled play. Gradually, he showed me more of himself but he remained frightened and ashamed of his feelings and thoughts and anxious that I would be disapproving or intrusive like his mum, so he often needed to shut me out.

Walking downstairs at the end of a silent session, he said: 'It's very dark and I'm going to die.' The next day he was reluctant to come to the room and then silently read a comic. After a while I said, 'I remember what you said yesterday. It was very important. You were really scared and couldn't tell me anything until you were leaving. Do you remember?' He said no. I tried again, 'I remember that you said it was very dark and you were going to die. It was such a scary feeling that you hardly dared to tell me. But you did, and that was very brave.' He said he didn't want to talk about it, but a bit later he said, 'When I'm in bed at night I worry about a war, about a bomb coming through the roof . . .

But I don't want to talk about it.' I reminded him that a few weeks ago he hadn't wanted to talk about his worry about going to the dentist, but he had been able to be brave enough to tell me and the talking had helped. 'Mm,' he said. 'It wasn't a worry about having my teeth pulled out.' We remembered that he'd been terrified that he would not wake up from the anaesthetic. 'Yes . . . I'm going to forget about it . . . But I can't . . . I keep dreaming about it. I dream that I'm a doctor doing that to someone else. It's better to do it to someone than have it done to you.' I said, 'Yes, imagining scaring and hurting someone else is a way of trying to manage the worry.'

The following day we played draughts. I said the game was a bit like a battle with two armies fighting. When he moved his white pieces, he used a baby voice to make the piece talk about moving forward but staying safe. Soon it became clear that he was playing out a fantasy in which the babies (his white pieces) were going to be killed by the grown-ups (my black pieces). In order to stay alive, the babies had to kill the murderous parents, but the babies were captured, put in prison and had their heads chopped off. As each baby was beheaded, it joined with another 'dead' baby until he ended up with one enormous white piece made up of all the previously 'dead' pieces. As the white piece increased in size, it became the 'king', then the 'queen', 'King Kong', the 'bla-bla monster', the 'double bla-bla monster', and finally the 'triple bla-bla monster'. It was all-powerful and stronger than all my black 'adult' pieces. I said: 'So, the biggest baby triple bla-bla monster in the whole world feels safe at last because no one can capture or kill him and he is powerful enough to kill all the parents.' Ben grinned with triumph. At the end of the session, he carefully put the counters in the box in pairs, but surprisingly with a black and a white one in each pair. I asked, 'Do some of the babies want to be back with their parents?' In a baby voice, he replied, 'Yes, but some don't.' I talked about the baby part of Ben feeling so scared and cross with his parents that he wanted to kill them – but that was such a scary thought that he imagined instead that *they* were murderers, but that was terrifying too. I said that all the killing feelings felt just too awful and he preferred to forget them all. 'Yes . . . like the bomb worry . . . it's the baby bit of me that gets very scared, and the big part tells the baby part it's safe and there are no wars and no bombs.'

Ben felt utterly overwhelmed by his aggressive impulses and anger towards his parents, especially mother, and consequently was afraid of separating from her. His massive defences against aggression severely restricted his life. Eventually, we discovered his phantasy that if he could be a girl or a baby he would be free of the turmoil of his anxiety and destructive aggression. Analysis of his fears, phantasies and defences (especially concerning aggression) enabled him to want to grow up into a man and freed him to enter a more typical and enjoyable latency.

Puberty and adolescence

At puberty, children are besieged by increasing sexual and aggressive forces as their bodies undergo massive physical and hormonal changes, giving rise to much anxiety and confusion. As their bodies mature, they face the excitement, responsibilities, fantasies and fears that accompany the approach of adulthood, including the reality that they will soon be as big, powerful and sexually active as the parents. This feels potentially exciting *and* lonely and terrifying. Pubertal children experience an enormous sense of loss of their childhood body image and of mother as their chief caretaker (Laufer 1981). Previously, they could rely on adults intervening if their aggression got out of hand, but their increased physical strength means taking further responsibility for the damage their body could do.

Adolescents typically struggle with the conflict of wishing to be looked after like a dependent child (regressive wishes which they also defend against) and wanting to become an independent adult (which they also fear). Alongside this, they struggle to find an identity that will make them feel good about themselves. To defend against fears of regression, dependence and passivity, they may develop a self-image of being invulnerable, independent and aggressive. Although this is more obvious in adolescent boys, for whom conflicts of passivity and dependence arouse age-typical homosexual anxieties, the following shows some of the roots of this conflict in an adolescent girl:

> At 18, Lisa had a breakdown at university. Her sado-masochistic style of relating had caused her to lose friends and boyfriends, but she apparently revelled in the image of herself as a 'tough, provocative bitch'. She was attempting to defend against conflicts over regression and dependence, and trying to find some kind of stable self-image in defiance of a sadistic superego that impatiently demanded perfection. Such a harsh superego undermined any good feelings about herself and she resorted to rebelling and giving free rein to her destructiveness as temporary means to raise her self-esteem. She said, 'If I feel depressed, I have to fight. It's the only way I know of relating to people and finding out if they care or not. Fighting and provoking are my best talents. I'm not good at anything else.'
>
> Consciously desperate for help, she started analysis five times a week, but her huge anxiety led to intense resistance. Terrified of separation and loss (though she denied this vehemently), she defended herself by not engaging with me or allowing herself to recognise any feelings of attachment. She often arrived 30 minutes late, or not at all, and was

quite contemptuous of me. She announced: 'Analysis is pointless anyway because I'm too crazy. Even a hundred Sigmund Freuds would never figure me out.' I addressed her despair that she was irreparably damaged and mad and interpreted her disappointment at being stuck with an ordinary therapist, not a celebrated 'ideal': if she could not be perfect, she felt worthless; and if I wasn't Freud, I was useless. My struggle to contain my resentment and wish to retaliate was alleviated when I understood her dismissive behaviour *towards* me as an aggressively passive into active defence against feeling rejected *by* me. She was provoking me to test if I would reject and abandon her. Thinking of her aggression as like that of a panicky toddler in a tantrum helped me to regain my empathy. I interpreted her provocations as her wish to see if I could survive her attacks without rejecting her, as her wish to engage me in an exciting battle to ward off feelings of depression and emptiness and as her way of keeping control over the analysis for fear of being helplessly dependent on me. It soon became clear that her entrenched sado-masochistic style of relating provided a defence against core complex anxieties of abandonment and engulfment (Glasser 1996), whereby she could maintain an optimal distance from, yet also a hold on the object. Her defiance towards her parents and me was reflected in an internal sado-masochistic battle between a punitive superego and her demanding and aggressive infantile wishes. Her aggression, directed towards others and herself via self-destructive and risk-taking behaviour, was insufficiently bound with loving feelings. She had no capacity for real concern – either for others or for herself. She felt spoilt by her parents 'as if they don't care' and swung between a deeply self-denigrating self-image and a view of herself, imbued with bravado, as omnipotent and grandiose.

During adolescence, some risky behaviour is expectable as teenagers test their limits and 'try on' different types of identity, but (as with Lisa) risk taking may represent an unresolved sense of omnipotence and the avoidance of independent mastery and self-care, developmental issues faced by the child in toddlerhood. A major developmental task of adolescence involves loosening the libidinal and aggressive ties to the parents in order to become an independent member of society. There are many reasons why an adolescent might be unable to detach in a healthy way from the parents, including unresolved ambivalence and aggression towards them. The adolescent may progress from suspiciousness of the parents to general paranoia. Or hostility and aggression may be deflected away from the parents and onto the self, leading to depression, self-denigration, self-harm and sometimes suicide.

Adolescence is a 'normative crisis situation' (Tonnesmann 1980) and a time of 'developmental disturbance' when the typical fluctuations 'between extreme opposites would be deemed highly abnormal at any other time of life' (Freud, A. 1980: 275). In the turmoil of adolescence, the young person's entire internal world is turned upside down. It is not surprising that they swing from wild excitement to deep depression and that their defences break down. Buxbaum wrote: 'Just as the river, swollen with melting snow and torrential rains, breaks through its dams and floods the land, so the inordinately increased aggression floods the adolescent's whole system, explodes, and inundates society' (Buxbaum 1970: 263). Delinquent and destructive enactments of aggression constitute the adolescent's rebellion not only against external authority but also, most importantly, against severe superego dictates. In the context of faulty superego development, guilt is unavailable as a signal and has to be defied and triumphed over.

Typical passions of the healthy adolescent concern matters of world importance – world peace, racism, animal rights – in their view, treated complacently by the adult world. Such ideals provide a focus for directing adolescent aggression and passions in very adaptive and socially useful ways, while also allowing them to feel superior to the parents as they individuate from them. If the adolescent's earlier development has been good enough, he will have established healthy modes of relating in which aggression is bound by loving and protective feelings so that aggression will be used for preservation of self and others and self-assertion. Physical aggression is sublimated through various hobbies, interests and skills and channelled into activities such as competitive sports and verbal debate and, fused with loving feelings, into sexual activity. Language becomes the major medium for the expression of aggression and, in the relatively healthy adolescent, this is confined to swearing and having the occasional row. The less healthy adolescent, who is still struggling to restrain his aggressive impulses, may be physically aggressive and will use words violently and destructively to vent his rage. This brings us back to the title of the chapter.

Conclusion

I began with 'biting teeth' and now end with 'biting wit', both aspects of oral aggression. If biting wit takes the form of sarcasm, the destructiveness remains undisguised, unfunny and potentially damaging. If, however, it takes the form of irony (such as political satire), the aggressive content and intent is less directly destructive. Thus channelled, it can be a source of pleasurable fun as well as a means of communicating an ideological view.

The development of aggression is a massive topic. Some aspects mentioned perhaps deserve greater emphasis, but I have aimed to trace the main normative developmental issues and to emphasise some of the positive aspects of aggression as these tend to be given less attention in the literature. A concluding quote from Anna Freud reminds us that we all retain traces of aggression from every developmental level, and that throughout our lives we continue to struggle with them:

> [W]hile libido and aggression move forward from one level to the next and cathect the objects which serve satisfaction on each stage, no station on the way is ever fully outgrown.
>
> (1980: 95)

Acknowledgements

In fond memory of Rose Edgcumbe for her wisdom and clarity of mind.

References

Blos, P. (1967) 'The second individuation process of adolescence', *Psychoanalytic Study of the Child* 22: 162–86

Bowlby, J. (1973) *Attachment and Loss, Vol. 2, Separation*, London: Hogarth Press
—— (1980) *Attachment and Loss, Vol. 3, Loss*, London: Hogarth Press

Buxbaum, E. (1970)'Aggression and the function of the group in adolescence' in *Troubled Children in a Troubled World*, New York: International Universities Press

Edgcumbe, R. (1976) 'The development of aggressiveness in children', *Nursing Times* 1 April (RCN Supplement): vii–xv

Edgcumbe, R. and Burgner, M. (1975) 'The phallic narcissistic phase: a differentiation between pre-oedipal and oedipal aspects of phallic development', *Psychoanalytic Study of the Child* 30: 161–80

Fraiberg, S. (1982) 'Pathological defences in infancy', *Psychoanalytic Quarterly* 51: 612–35

Freud, A. (1942) *The Ego and the Mechanisms of Defence*, London: Hogarth Press
—— (1949) 'Aggression in relation to emotional development: normal and pathological', *Psychoanalytic Study of the Child* 3/4: 37–42
—— (1958) 'Adolescence', *Psychoanalytic Study of the Child* 13: 255–78
—— (1972) 'Comments on aggression' in *Psychoanalytic Psychology of Normal Development*, London: Hogarth Press
—— (1980) *Normality and Pathology in Childhood: Assessments of Development*, London: Hogarth Press

Freud, S. (1920) 'Beyond the pleasure principle', *Standard Edition 18*, London: Hogarth Press
—— (1926) 'Inhibitions, symptoms and anxiety', *Standard Edition 20*, London: Hogarth Press

Furman, E. (1992) *Toddlers and their Mothers. A Study in Early Personality Development*, Madison, CT: International Universities Press

Glasser, M. (1996) 'Aggression and sadism in the perversions' in *Sexual Deviation*, 3rd edn, I. Rosen (ed.), Oxford: Oxford University Press

Heimann, P. and Valenstein, A. (1972) 'The psychoanalytical concept of aggression: an integrated summary', *International Journal of Psycho-Analysis* 53: 31–5

Hoffer, W. (1949) 'Mouth, hand, and ego-integration', *Psychoanalytic Study of the Child* 3/4: 49–56

Khan, M. (1973) 'The concept of cumulative trauma', *Psychoanalytic Study of the Child* 18: 286–306

Laufer, M.E. (1981) 'The adolescent's use of the body in object relationships and in the transference: a comparison of borderline and narcissistic modes of functioning', *Psychoanalytic Study of the Child* 36: 163–80

Parsons, M. and Dermen, S. (1999) 'The violent child and adolescent' in *The Handbook of Child and Adolescent Psychotherapy*, M. Lanyado and A. Horne (eds.), London: Routledge

Stern, D.N. (1985) *The Interpersonal World of the Human Infant*, New York: Basic Books

Tonnesmann, M. (1980) 'Adolescent re-enactment, trauma and reconstruction', *Journal of Child Psychotherpy* 6: 23–44

Winnicott, D.W. (1950–55) 'Aggression in relation to emotional development' in *Collected Papers: Through Paediatrics to Psychoanalysis*, London: Hogarth Press
—— (1963a) 'From dependence towards independence in the development of the individual' *The Maturational Processes and the Facilitating Environment*, London: Hogarth Press
—— (1963b) 'The development of the capacity for concern' in *The Maturational Processes and the Facilitating Environment*, London: Hogarth Press

Attachment, trauma and violence: understanding destructiveness from an attachment theory perspective

Paul Renn

Introduction

The social and political implications of aggression and destructiveness cannot be overstated. Violence in particular is seen by many as having reached epidemic proportions in modern society. A brief example from my forensic practice will help to make the point. After 20 years of marriage Michael battered his wife, Anna, to death with a claw hammer despite professing to love her. How is such an appallingly violent act to be understood? In attempting to answer this question, I later explore the case of Michael in greater detail from an attachment theory perspective. First, I summarize the main premises of attachment theory and the findings of attachment informed research that help to explicate male affective violence.

Attachment theory describes a behavioural system, the function of which is to regulate human attachment, exploration and fear. Attachment is defined as any form of behaviour that results in a person attaining and retaining proximity to a differentiated other (Bowlby 1980). Following Bowlby, I propose that the particular quality of love and security provided by the main caregiver helps the child to regulate the basic conflict between love and hate. Aggression and destructiveness are the result of traumatic disturbance of the infant–caregiver relationship. I contend that affective violence in particular is rooted in the disruption of processes of attachment and constitutes a disorganised maladaptive reaction to a perceived threat, or sense of endangerment, to the self. I argue that the meaning of a destructive act is to be discovered in the subject's particular relational matrix and that an understanding of such maladaptive behaviour is to be gained by attending to the person's phenomenological experience of unmourned loss and unresolved psychological trauma.

The dispute that arose between attachment theory and psychoanalysis some 50 years ago focused on what Bowlby saw as reluctance in analytic circles to examine the impact of real-life traumatic events in the genesis of pathology. Happily there are increasing signs of a rapprochement between attachment theory and psychoanalysis. This integrative process is given added impetus by neuroscientific research and studies into deprivation, trauma, affect regulation, dissociation and implicit-procedural memory. The findings of these various disciplines point to the central role of the infant–caregiver attachment relationship in the transmission and regulation of emotions and to the saliency of this intersubjective process to both brain development and cognitive mastery of experience. Attachment research suggests that the mind can continue to develop throughout the lifespan via changes in the internal working models of attachment.

Attachment theory and aggression

Pathological grief and mourning are at the centre of Bowlby's understanding of aggression and destructiveness in the context of the child's experience of separation and loss within the family. Loss may be experienced in numerous ways including threats of abandonment, parental rejection, depression, neglect and/or abuse (Bowlby 1979, 1988). In pathological mourning the child's unexpressed ambivalent feelings of yearning for, and anger with, the attachment figure are split off into a dissociated system of the personality and the loss is disavowed. Experience is structured, shaped and organised by characteristic patterns of interaction operating within the family's particular caregiving-attachment system giving rise to secure, insecure or disorganised patterns of attachment. These patterns are represented in internal working models of attachment, which tend to persevere into adulthood and serve to regulate, interpret and predict attachment-related behaviour, thoughts and feelings throughout the life cycle via the implicit-procedural memory system (Bowlby 1969; Schacter 1996; Schore 1994). Internal working models of attachment may be equated with internal object relationships.

Key to Bowlby's thinking on aggression is the evolutionary function of anger. Angry protest is an instinctive biological response to anxiety and fear of separation from the preferred attachment figure whose physical presence and emotional availability affords the child safety, protection and psychobiological regulation, thereby promoting exploratory behaviour (Bowlby 1969, 1973; Schore 1994). The adaptive function of anger is to increase the intensity of the communication to the lost person with the goal of achieving reunion. Proximity to the attachment figure re-establishes a sense of safety and security, together with the physiological modulation of the attachment, fear, and exploratory behavioural systems.

When the caregiver's emotional response to the infant's attachment signals is appropriate, sensitive and consistent, the child develops a secure pattern of attachment and the ability to gradually self-regulate negative affective states confident that care, comfort and soothing will be available at times of stress. The capacity for angry protest is healthy, indicating a secure attachment bond. When the caregiver's response is rejecting, inconsistent, or frightening, the infant develops an insecure or disorganised pattern of attachment. As a result the child is either inhibited about expressing protest and defiance or becomes locked into unassuaged aggression, developing mental models characterised by anger, mistrust, fear and hostility, together with maladaptive strategies for circumventing the perceived unresponsiveness of the attachment figure. This leaves the child vulnerable to psychopathology in later life.

When parents are unavailable and there is no substitute attachment figure, the child may move to a position of emotional detachment, defensively excluding attachment-related information from consciousness as a maladaptive means of suppressing dreaded psychobiological states of mind that threaten to overwhelm them. Bowlby (1980) regards defensive exclusion as constituting the heart of psychopathology because attachment-related behaviours, thoughts and feelings associated with the traumatic situation cease to be experienced. Consequently, the subject's cognitive-affective response to the loss or trauma becomes disconnected and the experience remains unprocessed. When the insecurely attached individual experiences separation and loss in adulthood, unresolved traumatic experiences may be activated, together with the dysfunctional expression of anger, hatred and hostility (Bowlby 1979, 1988). By contrast, the securely attached subject is guided by internal working models, enabling them to own and openly express appropriate anger and to contain and regulate aggressive feelings and destructive impulses when anger is aroused in situations involving pain and fear (Holmes 2001).

In sum, the caregiving environment generally and the infant–caregiver attachment relationship particularly initiate the child along one of an array of potential developmental pathways, with disturbance of attachment being the outcome of a series of deviations that take the child increasingly further from adaptive functioning. Internal working models of attachment provide the templates for psychopathology in later life, which may include aggressive and destructive forms of behaviour.

Contemporary views of trauma and affect regulation

Psychological trauma results in feelings of intense fear, helplessness and threat of annihilation, which disorganises mental functioning and overwhelms the adaptations that ordinarily provide people with a sense of control, emotional connection and meaning (Herman 1992). Traumatic affect is therefore viewed as a significant factor motivating aggression and destructiveness (DeZulueta 1993; Tyson & Tyson 1990). Bowlby's emphasis on the significance of the environment as a traumatic determinant of aggression appears to have been vindicated (Holmes 1993). However, when a child loses a parent, the damage sustained is caused not only by the loss itself but also by the attendant discord and disruption in the family (Rutter

1981). Moreover, the child may develop an attachment disorder in a stable, yet unhealthy, relationship (Rutter 1997). Disorganised unresolved states of mind develop when there are additional or interactive factors aggravating the traumatic event unless it falls 'well outside the norm' (Lyons-Ruth & Jacobvitz 1999: 547). The salient factor in personality development and adult psychopathology is the characteristic caregiving-attachment system within which the child experiences the trauma rather than the traumatic event itself (Renn 2003). These views indicate that *disorganisation* of the attachment relationship, rather than simply its insecurity, may be a central factor in the emergence of violence and aggression in later life.

Consideration of the impact of a traumatic event should include the effects of family dysfunction, parenting practices or parental psychopathology. Child abuse rarely occurs in isolation and its traumatic effects can often be explained by coexisting family dysfunction (Benjamin & Pugh 2001). Emotional abuse is more common and just as significant as physical or sexual abuse in the development of psychopathology because the child has to employ defensive strategies to deal with negative affect; for example, suppressing anger and sadness by being either good or inappropriately happy (Bradley 2003). The child's adaptive response to parental emotional abuse may be seen in terms of Winnicott's (1960) formulation of the false self.

An emerging body of evidence suggests that affect regulation constitutes an important part of the relationship between attachment and psychopathology (Bradley 2003). Affect regulation involves both appropriately dampening negative emotion and intensifying positive emotion, such as pride, joy and interest-excitement.

The caregiver's capacity to monitor and regulate their own negative affect plays a key role in regulating the child's affective states and in facilitating the child's ability to self-regulate emotion and therefore their sense of safety and security (Schore 1994). Attachment to the caregiver is promoted by the interactive regulation of emotion (Schore 1991, 1994, 2001). This intersubjective process involves recognising and labelling specific emotions in the self and in others and, optimally, the development of flexible strategies to control uncomfortable levels of arousal and to mediate interpersonal conflict (Bradley 2003).

In respect of the child's incapacity to modulate aggression, Schore (1991, 1994) implicates the caregiver's failure to interactively regulate negative affective states of fear, shame and rage during critical phases in the development of emotional systems in the right brain in the second year of life. Early unregulated shame exchanges, in particular, rupture the attachment bond and thus are important sources of severe emotional disorders associated with under-regulated aggression. Unregulated shame is 'bypassed' or dissociated by the child and later by the adult. This defensive manoeuvre inhibits exploration of the external environment and knowledge of internal emotional states, leading to an impaired ability to recognise, label and articulate discrete feeling states such as fear, distress and anger.

Relational trauma is typically embedded in the child's family situation and so is a cumulative event phenomenon. In cumulative relational trauma, the caregiver both dysregulates the infant's affective state and, crucially, either withholds any interactive repair or is inconsistent and ineffective in this endeavour. As a result of such severe misattunement the infant is left in an intensely disorganised psychobiological state, beyond their coping strategies. The infant's response to such a fear-inducing environment consists of hyper-vigilance and hyper-arousal, followed by hypo-arousal or dissociation, involving numbing, avoidance, compliance and restricted affect. The internalisation of such interactive patterns may interfere with the developing child's optimal regulation of arousal and compromise their capacity to stay attentive and process socio-emotional information, particularly when under heightened emotional stress.

The enduring effects of early relational trauma consist of a deficient capacity to process socio-emotional information and regulate bodily states. Disorganised attachment in particular produces maladaptive internal working models, leaving the individual vulnerable to affect dysregulation in interpersonal conflict situations (Bradley 2003). The dysregulation of fear states in early life results in permanent sensitivity to stress in adulthood because the subject cannot prevent an excessive reaction by terminating their stress response (Schore 2001). Traumatic early life events predispose certain individuals to later psychiatric disturbance when they re-experience an event matching the original stressor (Perry, Pollard, Blakely, Baker, & Vigilante 1995). An impaired ability to maintain interpersonal relationships, cope with stress, and regulate emotions is associated with anti-social and borderline personality disorders (Schore 1994). Informed by clinical experience, I argue that in many instances personality disorders may more appropriately be viewed as disorders of adult attachment.

The way in which the subject interprets traumatic and abusive experiences is central to the modulation of affective arousal and to the later development of symptoms and disorders (Herman & van der Kolk 1987; van der Kolk & Fisler 1995). Neuroscience research indicates that trauma induces a deficit in the brain's right orbitofrontal systems. As a result, affective information implicitly processed in the right brain is inefficiently transmitted to the left hemisphere for semantic processing (Schore 1994). Thus the psychological meaning of problematic emotional experience does not become organised into a coherent narrative and sense of self (Holmes 1999; Tyson & Tyson 1990). This increases the likelihood of the subject acting out impulsively or aggressively in situations of arousal (Bradley 2003; Schore 1994).

The resultant internal working models of attachment determine the individual's characteristic approach to affect regulation throughout life, being used as guides for future action. In essence, cumulative relational trauma in infancy, consisting of oscillating states of hyper-arousal and dissociation, becomes the template for adult post-traumatic stress disorder (Perry et al. 1995; Schore 1994). In such instances, substance misuse is often used as a means both of suppressing dreaded psychobiological states and of restoring a semblance of affect regulation.

Attachment theory and the transmission of affect

Attachment theory may be considered a theory of emotion regulation. The quality of caregiving transmits attachment organisation including a characteristic style of regulating affect. Subtle, fine-grain interactive microbehaviours are related to attachment and the transmission of emotion from one generation to the next (Beebe & Lachmann 1992; Peck 2003; Stern 1985). Such micro-behaviours operate at the level of implicit relational knowledge including the coordination of gaze direction, vocal inflections, body posture and facial expressions (Stern, Sander, Nahum, Harrison, Lyons-Ruth, Morgan, Bruschweiler-Stern & Tronick 1998). The infant perceives and remembers the mother's repetitive subtle behaviours. Thus, the cumulative impact of consistently matched or mismatched interactions creates a structuring effect on the infant who then generalises these expectancies to other interpersonal contexts.

Attachment research (Main 1991; Main, Kaplan, & Cassidy 1985), employing the adult attachment interview (George, Kaplan, & Main 1984) and the Strange Situation procedure (Ainsworth, Blehar, Waters, & Walls 1978), indicates that the parents' internal working models of attachment are transmitted to the growing child. These influence the child's working models of attachment, which in turn mediate all subsequent relationships, particularly with intimate partners in adulthood (Bowlby 1980; Holtzworth-Munroe, Stuart, & Hutchinson 1997; Roberts & Noller 1998). Caregivers with a secure style of attachment are skilled emotion regulators, capable of a wide range of emotional experience and expression (Peck 2003). They can observe their child's distress without becoming overly aroused by experiencing personal distress from their own attachment histories. The secure caregiver is free to respond to the infant's emotional distress in a flexible and appropriate manner, thereby repairing normal interactive ruptures to the attachment bond with relative consistency (Tronick, Als, Adams, Wise, & Brazelton 1978). The child, in turn, develops a matching secure pattern of attachment organisation and a free, flexible style of emotion regulation (Main et al. 1985).

Insecure patterns of attachment are transmitted to the infant by caregivers with either a predominantly dismissing or preoccupied style of attachment. In the former, the child's distress activates personal distress in the caregiver. The parent turns away from regulating the infant's stress, focusing instead on managing their own emotional conflicts. To avoid rejection, the child minimises expressions of need and vulnerability and becomes disconnected from his or her affective states. The preoccupied caregiver needs to have the child emotionally dependent on them and they focus on the infant's negative feelings instead of helping the child to regulate their emotions. This reduces the child's chances of becoming emotionally independent of the caregiver, and leads to an under-regulated style of modulating emotion, particularly anger (Main et al. 1985; Peck 2003).

Infants develop a disorganised pattern of attachment in reaction to caregivers who display frightened and frightening behaviour associated with their own unresolved early trauma. Such fear-inducing parental behaviour may constitute maltreatment or alternating forms of caregiving wherein emotional availability is followed by an abrupt entrance into dissociative states, activated by the child's distress and need of comfort. The child, in turn, comes to associate their own fearful arousal as a danger signal for abuse or abandonment (Main & Hesse 1990). In a caregiving-attachment system in which the infant's parent is both the source of fear and the only protective figure to whom to turn to resolve stress and anxiety, the child's attachment system remains in a state of high activation and they fail to develop a coherent strategy for coping with the stress of separation (Hesse & Main 2000; Lyons-Ruth & Jacobvitz 1999; Main & Hesse 1990). Repeated exposure to this paradoxical dilemma results in 'fright without solution' and a collapse of the child's organised attachment strategy, manifested as odd, disoriented approach-avoidant conflict behaviours. Since there is no physical escape from this traumatising situation, the infant shifts from states of hyper-arousal and angry protest to states of despair, followed by emotional detachment and dissociation, thereby matching the mother's dissociated state (Schore 1994, 2001).

Cumulative relational trauma has a negative impact on the infant's maturing right orbitofrontal system and can lead to a permanent dysregulation of fear states. This compromises brain-mediated functions such as attachment, empathy and affect regulation (Perry et al. 1995). Disorganised attachment during infancy shifts to controlling behaviour in the older child which may be expressed as a punitive style of relating or an overly solicitous compulsive form of caregiving (Solomon & George 1996). Disorganised attachment is associated with a predisposition to relational violence, to dissociative states and conduct disorders in children and adolescents and to borderline personality disorders in adults (Lyons-Ruth & Jacobvitz 1999). The rate of such disorders in forensic settings is particularly high (APA 1994; Hart 2001).

Dissociation disrupts the monitoring and attentional functions of consciousness making the person impervious to attachment communications and interactive regulation (Main 1991). Disorganised attachment and its attendant dissociation and dysregulated affect, constitutes a primary risk factor for the development of borderline and sociopathic personality disorders (Schore 1994). Clinically, dissociated experience is unsymbolised by thought and language, existing within the personality as a separate reality, cut off from authentic human relatedness (Bromberg 1998).

Separation and psychological differentiation

The provision by the caregiver of a secure base or safe haven facilitates the child's separation and exploration. Implicit in attachment theory, therefore, is the ability to separate while remaining attached. The child's sense of 'felt security' in relation to the main attachment figure vitally affects their freedom to explore the environment and elaborate and express their emotional states without becoming overly fearful (Sroufe & Waters 1977). Bowlby (1969) emphasises the ambivalent conflict between emotional connection and separateness, construing it as 'attachment and the dance with independence'.

Object relations (Balint 1979; Khan 1979; Winnicott 1960, 1974) and ego psychology (Mahler & Furer 1969) emphasise that the child needs a degree of aggression and defiance to attain an optimal sense of separateness and differentiation and thus to engage in autonomous exploration as an agentic self. Without difference there can be no subjective perspective (Benjamin 1992; Ogden 1986). Defiance and rebellion against parental authority tend to re-emerge in adolescence during what Blos terms 'the second individuation process' (1962: 77). Parental abuse, narcissism and neglect generate anxiety and insecurity, making separation and psychological differentiation problematic. The role of the father in helping the child to separate from a disturbed dyadic relationship with the mother is a vital aspect of the child's relational experience (Campbell 1999). The perspective of the father as a third object may provide the child with a second chance to develop a secure psychological self (Fonagy & Target 1999).

The frontal lobe areas of the brain integrate basic emotional processes with the ability for cognitive reflection (Panksepp 2001). This developmental process promotes the gradual emergence of the capacity for self-regulation and self-restraint, together with the ability to communicate effectively and share emotional experience with others (Panksepp 2001; Schore 1994, 2001; Siegal 2001; Trevarthen 2001). More fundamentally, children deprived of opportunities for rough and tumble games – a robust form of playful interaction typical of the child–father relationship – may exhibit slower neuronal maturation of the frontal lobes, a developmental delay associated with emotional and behavioural problems, particularly attention deficit and hyperactivity disorder (Panksepp 2001).

Despite their importance to the child's overall development, the father figure is often largely absent or emotionally unavailable. This factor is exacerbated by the excessive hours worked by many men and by the high rate of separation and divorce in contemporary western society. When the child's attachment to both parents is severely disturbed a developmental pathway leading to serious psychopathology is likely unless a buffering, protective effect is afforded by a secure attachment to at least one member of the child's family, for example, an aunt or grandparent (Holmes 2001). A meaningful attachment relationship provides the intersubjective basis for the development of the capacity to mentalise and, thereby, to reflect on and resolve traumatic and abusive experience (Fonagy et al. 1997). In such instances, the child who has been subjected to persistent parental maltreatment may be diverted from a developmental pathway that otherwise might culminate in borderline personality disorder.

Attachment theory and violence

Before discussing the link between attachment theory and interpersonal violence a distinction between violence and aggression may be helpful (DeZulueta 1993). Aggression may be defined as an attitude and style of relating to the other informed by anger, envy, hatred and hostility. Aggressive feelings and impulses may be expressed verbally, or be communicated non-verbally but unless acted out physically, do not constitute violence. By contrast, a violent act consists of an attack on the body of another with the explicit intention of causing physical harm and injury.

Violence falls into two broad types of behaviour: predatory or psychopathic violence, which is held to be planned and emotionless, in which the perpetrator seeks out a victim with whom he has no attachment relationship; and defensive or affective violence, which arises in reaction to a perceived threat to one's personal safety or sense of self, which is preceded by heightened levels of emotional arousal (Fonagy 1999; Gilligan 2000). Cartwright (2002) concurs with this distinction, but in line with Fonagy's (1999) conceptualisation of mentalisation, argues that both types of violence involve the expression of unbearable states of mind that cannot be reflected on or symbolised. In this chapter, I focus primarily on affective or defensive violence.

The most serious violent crime is homicide, which includes murder, manslaughter and infanticide. In England and Wales in 2002/2003 there were 1048 deaths recorded as homicide, many of which relate to women and children killed in a family situation. Home Office research estimates that in the same period there were 2.7 million violent incidents of varying degrees of seriousness involving adults (Povey & Allen 2003); and in 1995 there were 6.6 million incidents of domestic physical assaults (Mirrlees-Black 1999). Findings confirm that the vast majority of violent assaults between adults occur within an existing attachment relationship and fall into the defensive or affective category (Meloy 1992). Further, research shows that childhood physical and sexual abuse takes place mainly within a domestic situation and is perpetrated by a member of the child's family (Cawson, Watton, Brooker, & Kelly 2000).

In addressing human violence, Bowlby (1973, 1988) again emphasises that anger serves to maintain vitally important relationships and that violence may be understood as the distorted and exaggerated version of potentially functional attachment behaviour. Liotti (1992) connects disorganised attachment and dissociation with the construction of a multiple, incoherent mental model of the main attachment figure, contending that incompatible multiple models in respect of the same person generate oscillating beliefs and expectations. At times of intense emotional stress the earlier, less conscious, models tend to become dominant. In later life, separations and losses may activate confused, unstable cognitive-affective models, imbued with dysregulated rage and fury deriving from childhood fear of abandonment, shame, and dread of loneliness, resulting in extreme behaviour, including violence (Bowlby 1973, 1979).

Bowlby (1988) suggests that murder may often be explained by the perpetrator's inability to tolerate the attachment figure leaving. This contention seems to be confirmed by data showing that spousal murder, imbued with intense affective violence, is most likely to occur immediately after physical separation (Dutton 1995; Mirrlees-Black 1999). Bradley (2003) cites findings demonstrating an association between separation distress and elevated secretions of cortisol, a negative neurochemical. She argues that together, these factors overwhelm the limited coping strategies of the insecurely attached individual. Neuroimaging research has found reduced prefrontal and increased subcortical brain activity in both predatory and affective murderers, indicating that a reduction in right orbitofrontal functioning may be particularly implicated in a predisposition to violence (Raine, Meloy, Bihrle, Stoddard, Lacasse, & Buchsbaum 1998).

Comparative studies of violent offenders reveal that some men who kill present as 'normal', even model citizens whose early environments seem to have been relatively benign. In such cases, the violent act and the accompanying affective rage, appears to be sudden and inexplicable, arising in response to little or no provocation (Cartwright 2002; Weiss, Lamberti, & Blackman 1960). Fonagy and Target (1999) postulate that in these cases the violent individual's psychological self has been violated in childhood in more subtle and covert ways than in those involving overt trauma and abuse. I concur with this contention and argue that the very normality of the violent man constitutes an aspect of a complex, but rigid, defensive organisation forged in a caregiving-attachment system characterised by subtle relational trauma that is cumulative in its effect (see p.63). In my clinical experience, the 'normal' murderer has remained psychologically merged with his early objects and therefore lacks the security to exist as a separate, autonomous self. This generates existential anxiety and internal conflict between fear of engulfment and fear of abandonment. I argue that a central aspect of the 'normal' murderer's defensive structure consists of a false-self organisation whose compliant, acquiescent behaviour and attitude of 'pseudo-independence' are reinforced by emotional detachment, idealisation and a 'moral defence'. Without a sense of internal security, the person perceives himself as bad in order to keep those on whom he depends for external security as good, despite, at times, experiencing his objects as tantalising and deeply disappointing (Fairbairn 1943). Thus, for defensive reasons, pain and distress are disavowed and good and bad aspects of the self are encapsulated in split-off parts of the personality. Negative affective states imbued with fear, shame, rage and hate are dissociated because they are experienced as too terrifying to face (Fairbairn 1943; Winnicott 1958, 1960). Anger, anxiety and ambivalent feelings of love and hate are warded off, in part by controlling the partner's emotional availability, either by avoidance of intimacy or by a compulsive form of caregiving.

These maladaptive styles of attachment behaviour are motivated by conflicting states of fear oscillating between engulfment and abandonment. The individual is able to modulate normative levels of stress and emotional arousal and may attain considerable success in career and financial terms. However, when rejected and abandoned by his partner and separated from children of the created family, exacerbated by stressful factors, such as sexual jealousy, bereavement, redundancy and financial problems, the person's conscious coping strategies and unconscious defensive structure break down. This activates a multiple disorganised internal working model and a maladaptive incoherent response, culminating in the enactment of a long suppressed, shame-driven explosive rage deriving from the original traumatising relational matrix in which the self was felt to be endangered.

Adult affective violence is rooted in disorganised attachment linked to unresolved trauma and to a dissociated representational system characterised by dysregulated affect and pathological mourning. The violent male feels trapped and helpless in the traumatising situation: fearing both abandonment and intimacy, he lacks the freedom to act as an agentic self and the capacity to develop a secure attachment relationship. At the moment of assault his over-controlled attachment system and tenuous capacity for mentalisation are overwhelmed by negative affect and distorted perceptions deriving from his personal trauma and re-experienced as an imminent threat to the self (Renn 2003; West & George 1999).

Figure 4.1 details the theoretical model that I have developed to explicate male affective violence and Figure 4.2 depicts my therapeutic model for working with violent men. Although the latter figure indicates a linear therapeutic progression, in practice, there is considerable interweaving of the clinical issues as these are worked on in an intersubjective process with the violent individual. While this attachment-based psychodynamic model has emerged from my work with violent men, I have found it to be equally effective in private practice with non-forensic clients of both genders whose

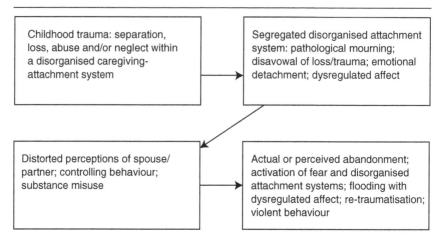

Figure 4.1 Relationship of childhood trauma to affective male violence in adulthood

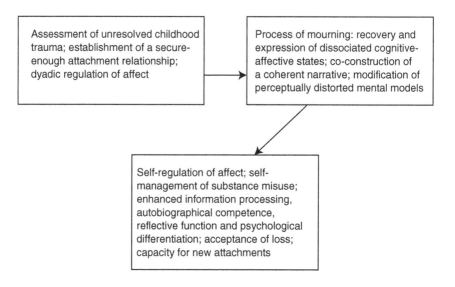

Figure 4.2 Conceptual structure of the proposed therapeutic model

destructive and self-destructive behaviours derive from early disorganised attachments and unprocessed experience associated with loss, abuse and trauma.

With regard to gender differences and violent behaviour, Mirrlees-Black (1999) found relatively similar levels of domestic violence for both men and women; the injuries inflicted on women by men, however, were more serious, reflecting their greater physical strength. Although the incidence of violence by women in the public domain is increasing, Roberts and Noller (1998) cite research which shows that, when compared to violent men, violent women are not violent outside their marital relationships. The authors suggest that attachment insecurity underlies women's use of violence and that such insecurity arises in the private domain as the couple struggle to manage their respective attachment conflicts over discomfort with closeness and fear of abandonment.

A clinical vignette from forensic practice

In clinical practice, attachment theory is used to conceptualise the developmental antecedents and interpersonal features of the client's problems, particularly their strategy for managing closeness and distance in intimate relationships and the influence of these factors on the formation of the therapeutic alliance (Lopez & Brennan 2000). As Slade (1999) notes, attachment theory and research provide a particular way of listening to the client's story and understanding the clinical process. Part of this process involves identifying similarities in the complex dynamic interplay between the client's early relational matrix and their current intimate relationships, including that with the therapist. This facilitates understanding how archaic cognitive-affective working models of attachment are perpetuated in the present, particularly at times of heightened emotional stress.

From an attachment theory perspective, the client's symptoms and destructive behaviour are understood as expressing unprocessed traumatic experience imprinted in implicit-procedural memories, as represented in self–other internal working models. These affective memories and interactional patterns emerge in the relational system or intersubjective field and are communicated directly to the therapist by the client's expressive behavioural display, which activates or elicits a matching countertransferential response in the therapist (Litowitz 2002; Orange 1995; Westen & Gabbard 2002).

The case of Michael, with which I opened this chapter, illustrates salient theoretical points, particularly the way in which loss, abuse and trauma are implicated in developmental pathways that culminate in violent, aggressive and destructive forms of behaviour. Names have been changed and personal circumstances disguised in order to protect identities.

Michael

Michael killed his estranged wife, Anna, hitting her head repeatedly with a claw hammer in an explosive rage after confronting her about the 'accusations she was making about me to the children'. He was 49 at the time and had been married to Anna for 20 years with four children aged 10 to 18 years.

Michael's parents separated when he was aged 4. He soon lost contact with his father after his mother re-married. He became estranged from his mother when she and his stepfather became preoccupied with running a small business and he developed a substitute attachment with his maternal grandmother, since she was now chiefly responsible for his upbringing. Michael had nothing in common with his stepfather and their relationship was distant and strained. His relationships with his parents deteriorated further when his half-sister was born because he felt they favoured her over him. This situation seemed to reinforce Michael's sense of rejection and foster a nascent misogynistic attitude. At about that time his grandfather's friend sexually abused him. He frequently ran away from home and suffered from persistent enuresis. He had six months' therapy with a child psychiatrist.

In early adulthood Michael became engaged to Clare, who precipitously broke off the engagement. On subsequently meeting Clare by chance they argued and Michael stabbed her in the chest. He was convicted of grievous bodily harm (GBH) and imprisoned. On his release a spate of offending behaviour occurred, culminating in a four-year sentence of imprisonment for offences of robbery, possession of a firearm and GBH with intent. Michael's criminal activity ceased following his marriage to Anna. In the four years prior to his killing her tension mounted in the marriage. He was working long, unsocial hours and Anna suspected him of having an extra-marital affair. They led increasingly separate lives, rarely having sex and frequently arguing. Their problems were exacerbated by Anna's excessive drinking and his controlling behaviour. Michael's grandmother and mother both died at that time causing him intense distress. He was reluctant to share the money he inherited with Anna because he suspected that she would use it to 'leave me'.

The couple tried but failed to reconcile their differences. Michael was hospitalised with depression after a suicide attempt. Within two weeks of being discharged, Anna accused him of raping her and he was arrested and remanded in custody for three months. During his time on remand Anna filed for divorce. Four days after his release he went to see Anna and killed her when she refused to talk to him, attempted to phone the police and flee from the house. Afterwards Michael explained that 'all my anger and frustration suddenly burst out'. The police were called and found Michael sitting in his car outside the family home. He was convicted of manslaughter and sentenced to seven years' imprisonment.

Michael spoke of loving Anna and of not wanting them to separate and divorce. However, he felt she provoked him by alleging rape, by tarnishing his name with their children, by withdrawing sexually from him and by planning to divorce him, leaving him shamed and humiliated in her, and the children's, eyes. Michael seemed emotionally detached and unable to empathise with Anna but he was deeply distressed by 'the grief I've caused my children' when he had wanted to give them the 'perfect childhood I didn't have'.

Setting aside his cumulative relational trauma, and the effect of this on his neurological development, Michael's formative experiences consisted of overt trauma in the form of loss, broken attachments and sexual abuse. In the absence of appropriate help to process these experiences, he developed a disorganised pattern of attachment and concomitant difficulty in regulating negative emotional states associated with rejection and abandonment. In childhood, he expressed his anger and distress by running away from home and bedwetting, whereas in adulthood it was enacted in violent crime. His secure-enough attachment to Anna enabled Michael to contain his fear and anxiety and his offending behaviour ceased. However, it appears that he defended against unresolved childhood trauma by controlling Anna and idealising the relationships with his children. While Anna was emotionally available to him such defences and coping strategies kept his fear and anxiety within manageable proportions. However, perceiving that Anna was intent on leaving him activated Michael's fear and attachment systems. His behaviour became increasingly disorganised and his coping strategies and mental defences were overwhelmed by dysregulated negative affect, resulting in an explosive murderous rage. His attack on Clare, when she rejected and abandoned him, may also be seen as indicating that loss triggered multiple incoherent internal working models, deriving from disorganised attachment to his early caregivers. Michael's anger and violence may thus be understood as a pathological form of attachment behaviour motivated by fear and the urgent need to protect the self from being re-traumatised.

Given Michael's lack of a coherent strategy to deal with separation, I considered it probable that any woman with whom he developed an intimate relationship would be at risk of harm when the relationship broke up. I reasoned that engaging him in work informed by an attachment-based psychodynamic approach would ameliorate his catastrophic experience of loss, rejection and abandonment and thereby reduce the risk to women in the future. Tragically, the opportunity did not arise. Later I heard that Michael had become intimately involved with a woman and battered her to death when she wanted to end the relationship. He went on the run after leaving a note admitting to killing her and directing the police to her body.

Conclusion

In this chapter, I have presented an attachment theory perspective to understanding aggression and destructiveness. In developing my argument, I have emphasised the relationships between trauma, disorganised attachment, affect regulation and psychopathology in adulthood, particularly interpersonal violence. I have proposed that vulnerability to stress derives, in large part, from cumulative relational trauma in early development within a particular caregiving-attachment system, and that fear and intense stress overwhelms the individual's conscious coping strategies and unconscious defensive structure. I have suggested that personality disorders may often be synonymous with disorders of adult attachment and I have illustrated theoretical points with a clinical case vignette. Finally, I have proposed a therapeutic model that recognises the importance of helping individuals to regulate their traumatic affective states within a secure-enough therapeutic relationship.

Acknowledgements and disclaimer

The author would like to thank the editor and Gwen Adshead, Sue Egan, Bernice Laschinger, Lynda Morgan, Joseph Schwartz and Kate White for their support and helpful comments in preparing this chapter for publication.

The views expressed in this chapter are solely those of the author and do not represent the views of the National Probation Service.

References

Ainsworth, M., Blehar, M., Waters, E. and Walls, S. (1978) *Patterns of Attachment: Assessed in the Strange Situation and at Home*, Hillsdale, NJ: Lawrence Erlbaum

American Psychiatric Association (1994) *Diagnostic and Statistical Manual of Mental Disorders*, 4th edn, Washington, DC: American Psychiatric Association

Balint, M. (1979) *The Basic Fault*, London: Routledge

Beebe, B. and Lachmann, F.M. (1992) 'The contribution of mother–infant mutual influence to the origins of self- and object representations' in *Relational Perspectives in Psychoanalysis*, N.J. Skolnick and S.C. Warshaw (eds), Hillsdale, NJ: The Analytic Press

Benjamin, J. (1992) 'Recognition and destruction: an outline of intersubjectivity' in *Like Subjects, Love Objects: Essays on Recognition and Sexual Difference*, New Haven, CT: Yale University Press

Benjamin, L.S. and Pugh, C. (2001) 'Using interpersonal theory to select effective treatment interventions' in *Handbook of Personality Disorders: Theory, Research, and Treatment*, W.J. Livesley (ed.), New York: The Guilford Press

Blos, P. (1962) 'The second individuation process of adolescence' in *On Adolescence: A Psychoanalytic Interpretation*, London: Free Association Books

Bowlby, J. (1969) *Attachment and Loss, Vol. 1: Attachment*, London: Pimlico

—— (1973) *Attachment and Loss, Vol. 2: Separation: Anger and Anxiety*, London: Pimlico

—— (1979) *The Making and Breaking of Affectional Bonds*, London: Routledge

—— (1980) *Attachment and Loss, Vol. 3: Loss: Sadness and Depression*, London: Pimlico

—— (1988) *A Secure Base: Clinical Applications of Attachment Theory*, Bristol: Arrowsmith

Bradley, S.J. (2003) *Affect Regulation and the Development of Psychopathology*, New York: The Guilford Press

Bromberg, P.M. (1998) *Standing in the Spaces: Essays on Clinical Process, Trauma and Dissociation*, Hillsdale, NJ: The Analytic Press

Campbell, D. (1999) 'The role of the father in a pre-suicide state' in *Psychoanalytic Understanding of Violence and Suicide*, R.S. Perelberg (ed.), London: Routledge

Cartwright, D. (2002) *Psychoanalysis, Violence and Rage-Type Murder: Murdering Minds*, Hove: Brunner-Routledge

Cawson, P., Watton, C., Brooker, S. and Kelly, G. (2000) *Child Maltreatment in the United Kingdom*, London: NSPCC Publications

DeZulueta, F. (1993) *From Pain to Violence: The Traumatic Roots of Destructiveness*, London: Whurr

Dutton, D. (1995) *The Domestic Assault of Women*, Vancouver: University of British Columbia Press

Fairbairn, W.R.D. (1943) 'The repression and return of bad objects (with special reference to the "war neuroses"' in *Psychoanalytic Studies of the Personality*, D.E. Scharff and E. Fairbairn Birtles (eds), London: Routledge

Fonagy, P. (1999) 'The male perpetrator: the role of trauma and failures of mentalization in aggression against women – an attachment theory perspective', unpublished paper given at the 6th John Bowlby Memorial Lecture, London, 20th February

Fonagy, P. and Target, M. (1999) 'Towards understanding violence: the use of the body and the role of the father' in *Psychoanalytic Understanding of Violence and Suicide*, R.S. Perelberg (ed.), London: Routledge

Fonagy, P., Target, M., Steele, M., Steele, H., Leigh, T., Levinson, A. and Kennedy, R. (1997) 'Morality, disruptive behaviour, borderline personality disorder, crime, and their relationships to security of attachment' in *Attachment and Psychopathology*, L. Atkinson and K.J. Zucker (eds), New York: The Guilford Press

George, C., Kaplan, N. and Main, M. (1984) Adult attachment interview, 1st edn, unpublished manuscript, Department of Psychology, University of California at Berkeley

Gilligan, J. (2000) *Violence: Reflections on Our Deadliest Epidemic*, London: Jessica Kingsley

Hart, S.D. (2001) 'Forensic issues' in *Handbook of Personality Disorders: Theory, Research, and Treatment*, New York: The Guilford Press

Herman, J.L. (1992) *Trauma and Recovery*, New York: Basic Books

Herman, J.L. and van der Kolk, B.A. (1987) 'Traumatic antecedents of borderline personality disorder' in *Psychological Trauma*, B.A. van der Kolk (ed.), Washington, DC: American Psychiatric Press

Hesse, E. and Main, M. (2000) 'Disorganized infant, child and adult attachment: collapse in behavioural and attentional strategies', *Journal of the American Psychoanalytic Association* 48: 1097–127

Holmes, J. (1993) *John Bowlby and Attachment Theory*, London: Routledge

—— (1999) 'Defensive and creative uses of narrative in psychotherapy: an attachment theory perspectives' in *Healing Stories: Narrative in Psychiatry and Psychotherapy*, G. Roberts and J. Holmes (eds), Oxford: Oxford University Press

—— (2001) *The Search for the Secure Base: Attachment Theory and Psychotherapy*, Hove; Brunner-Routledge

Holtzworth-Munroe, A., Stuart, G.L. and Hutchinson, G. (1997) 'Violent versus nonviolent husbands: differences in attachment patterns, dependency, and jealousy', *Journal of Family Psychology* 11(3): 314–31

Khan, M. (1979) *Alienation in Perversions*, London: Karnac

Liotti, G. (1992) 'Disorganized/disoriented attachment in the etiology of the dissociative disorders', *Dissociation* 4: 196–204

Litowitz, B.E. (2002) 'Sexuality and textuality', *Journal of the American Psychoanalytic Association* 50(1): 171–98

Lopez, F.G. and Brennan, K.A. (2000) 'Dynamic processes underlying adult attachment organization: toward an attachment perspective on the healthy and effective self', *Journal of Counseling Psychology* 47(3): 283–300

Lyons-Ruth, K. and Jacobvitz, D. (1999) 'Attachment disorganization: unresolved loss, relational violence and lapses in behavioural and attentional strategies' in *Handbook of Attachment: Theory, Research and Clinical Applications*, J. Cassidy and P.R. Shaver (eds), New York: The Guilford Press

Mahler, M.S. and Furer, M. (1969) 'On human symbiosis and the vicissitudes of individuation: infantile psychosis', *Journal of the American Psychoanalytic Association* 15: 740–53

Main, M. (1991) 'Metacognitive knowledge, metacognitive monitoring, and singular (coherent) vs multiple (incoherent) models of attachment: findings and directions for future research' in *Attachment Across the Life Cycle*, C.M. Parkes, J. Stevenson-Hinde and P. Marris (eds), London: Routledge

Main, M. and Hesse, E. (1990) 'Parents' unresolved traumatic experiences are related to infant disorganized attachment status: is frightened and/or frightening parental behaviour the linking mechanism?' in *Attachment in the Preschool Years: Theory, Research and Intervention*, M. Greenberg, D. Cicchetti, and E.M. Cummings (eds), Chicago: University of Chicago Press

Main, M., Kaplan, N. and Cassidy, J. (1985) 'Security in infancy, childhood, and adulthood: a move to the level of representation' in *Growing Points in Attachment: Theory and Research*, I. Bretherton and E. Waters (eds), Monographs of the Society for Research in Child Development. Chicago: University of Chicago Press

Meloy, J.R. (1992) *Violent Attachments*, London: Jason Aronson

Mirrlees-Black, C. (1999) *Domestic Violence: Findings from a New British Crime Survey Self-completion Questionnaire*, London: Home Office

Ogden, T.H. (1986) *The Matrix of the Mind: Object Relations and the Psychoanalytic Dialogue*, Northvale, NJ: Jason Aronson

Orange, D.M. (1995) *Emotional Understanding: Studies in Psychoanalytic Epistemology*, New York: The Guilford Press

Panksepp, J. (2001) 'The long-term psychobiological consequences of infant emotions: prescriptions for the twenty-first century', *Infant Mental Health Journal* 22: 132–73

Peck, S.D. (2003) 'Measuring sensitivity moment-by-moment: a micro analytic look at the transmission of affect', *Journal of Attachment and Human Development* 5(1): 38–63

Perry, B.D., Pollard, R.A., Blakely, T.L., Baker, W.L. and Vigilante, D. (1995) 'Childhood trauma, the neurobiology of adaptation, and "use-dependent" development of the brain. How "states" become "traits"', *Infant Mental Health Journal* 16: 271–91

Povey, D. and Allen, J. (2003) 'Violent crime in England and Wales' in *Violent Crime in England and Wales 2002/2003*, J. Simmons and T. Dodd (eds), London: Home Office

Raine, A., Meloy, J.R., Bihrle, S., Stoddard, J., Lacasse, L. and Buchsbaum, M.S. (1998) 'Reduced prefrontal and increased subcortical brain functioning assessed using positron emission tomography in predatory and affective murderers', *Behavioural Sciences and the Law* 16: 319–32

Renn, P. (2003) 'The link between childhood trauma and later violent offending: the application of attachment theory in a probation setting' in *A Matter of Security: The Application of Attachment Theory to Forensic Psychiatry and Psychotherapy*, F. Pfäfflin and G. Adshead (eds), London: Jessica Kingsley

Roberts, N. and Noller, P. (1998) 'The associations between adult attachment and couple violence: the role of communication patterns and relationship satisfaction' in *Attachment and Close Relationships*, J. Simpson and S. Rholes (eds), New York: The Guilford Press

Rutter, M. (1981) *Maternal Deprivation Reassessed*, 2nd edn, Harmondsworth: Penguin

—— (1997) 'Clinical implications of attachment concepts. Retrospective and prospective' in *Attachment Psychopathology*, L. Atkinson and K.J. Zucker (eds), New York: The Guilford Press

Schacter, D.L. (1996). *Searching for Memory: The Brain, the Mind, and the Past*, New York: Basic Books

Schore, A.N. (1991) 'Early superego development: the emergence of shame and narcissistic affect regulation in the practicing period', *Psychoanalysis and Contemporary Thought* 14: 187–250

—— (1994) *Affect Regulation and the Origin of the Self: The Neurobiology of Emotional Development*, Hillsdale, NJ: Lawrence Erlbaum

—— (2001) 'The effects of early relational trauma on right brain development, affect regulation, and infant mental health', *Infant Mental Health Journal* 22: 201–69

Siegal, D.J. (2001) 'Toward an interpersonal neurology of the developing mind: attachment relationships, "mindsight" and neural integration', *Infant Mental Health Journal* 22: 67–94

Slade, A. (1999) 'Attachment theory and research: implications for the theory and practice of individual psychotherapy with adults' in *Handbook of Attachment: Theory, Research and Clinical Applications*, J. Cassidy and P.R. Shaver (eds), New York: The Guilford Press

Solomon, J. and George, C. (1996) 'Defining the caregiving system: toward a theory of caregiving', *Infant Mental Health Journal* 17: 183–97

Sroufe, L.A. and Waters, E. (1977) 'Attachment as an organizational construct', *Child Development* 48: 1184–99

Stern, D.N. (1985) *The Interpersonal World of the Infant: A View from Psychoanalysis and Developmental Psychology*, New York: Basic Books

Stern, D.N., Sander, L.W., Nahum, J.P., Harrison, A.M., Lyons-Ruth, K., Morgan, A.C., Bruschweiler-Stern, N. and Tronick, E.Z. (1998) 'The process of therapeutic change involving implicit knowledge: some implications of developmental observations for adult psychotherapy', *Infant Mental Health Journal* 19(3): 300–8

Trevarthen, C. (2001) 'Intrinsic motives for companionship in understanding: their origin, development, and significance for infant mental health', *Infant Mental Health Journal* 22: 95–131

Tronick, E., Als, H., Adams, L., Wise, S. and Brazelton, T.B. (1978) 'The infant's response to entrapment between contradictory messages in face-to-face interaction', *Journal of American Child Psychiatry* 17: 1–13

Tyson, P. and Tyson, R.L. (1990) *Psychoanalytic Theories of Development: An Integration*, New Haven, CT: Yale University Press

van der Kolk, B.A. and Fisler, R. (1995) 'Dissociation and the fragmentary nature of traumatic memories: overview and exploratory study', *Journal of Traumatic Stress* 8(4): 505–21

Weiss, J., Lamberti, J. and Blackman, N. (1960) 'The sudden murderer: a comparative analysis', *Archives of General Psychiatry* 2: 669–78

West, M. and George, C. (1999) 'Abuse and violence in intimate adult relationships: new perspectives from attachment theory', *Journal of Attachment and Human Development* 1(2): 137–156

Westen, D. and Gabbard, G.O. (2002) 'Developments in cognitive neuroscience: II. implications for theories of transference', *Journal of the American Psychoanalytic Association* 50(1): 99–134

Winnicott, D.W. (1958) 'The capacity to be alone', *International Journal of Psycho-Analysis* 39: 416–20

—— (1960) 'Ego distortion in terms of true and false self' in *Maturational Processes and the Facilitating Environment*, London: Hogarth Press

—— (1974) 'Fear of breakdown', *International Journal of Psycho-Analysis* 1: 103–7

'In pieces': the effects of the memory of a violent father on a son's development

Anne Harrison

Introduction

As psychoanalysis has evolved, so too has the range and focus of our understanding of the role of the father in psychic development and the structuring of the self. In Freud's account of sexual development (1916–17), the Oedipus Complex and the child's recognition of genital difference serve to bind and structure the fluid possibilities of the pre-genital era and establish sexual identity and a choice of object. The oedipal father threatens castration and bears an authority that, once internalised, installs his son, at any rate, in a secure relationship with both reality and the moral order (Freud 1923). Within this frame of reference, the image of the mother seems benign and oddly generalised.

As new generations of analytic thinkers began to address the intricacies of early psychic life, however, the complexity of the child's relationship with the pre-oedipal mother became apparent. Recognition of the ambiguity, intensities and ambivalence of this relationship brought a new layer of significance to the role of the father. Where the developmental task is seen as 'psychic hatching' from a primary mother–infant matrix, fathers play a crucial part, aiding and consolidating the emerging separation from mother, long before the struggles of oedipality begin. In a key paper Leowald (1951) describes the importance of father as a second object, distinct from mother, with whom the child identifies in a way that nourishes and protects his emerging sense of self. Psychic representation of the father allows for triangulation, which eases the ricochet of projections in the infant–mother dyad (Lebovici 1982) and assists the child's emergence from it (Greenspan 1982). Gaddini (1982) writes subtly of the father as the first external object and of the triangular situation that serves to establish mother properly as an object and not just a part of the 'infant's' self-experience.

An important contribution was made to the discussion by French analysts, from Lacan (1964) onwards, who emphasised that it is the representation of father carried in the mother's mind that is significant for psychic development (McDougall 1989), as well as the part played by representations of the parents in relation to one another (Laplanche & Pontalis 1973). In a fascinating account of the oedipal moment, Britton (1989) uses the theme of representation of the parental couple to argue that it is only when an image of parents as a couple in a loving connection has been internalised that an individual becomes fully separate and capable of self-reflection. From a clinical study of work with 13 children with absent fathers, Burgner (1985) confirmed the importance of a second object – father or therapist – in reinforcing the sense of boundary and differentiation from mother and freeing the child from the toils of primitive, dyadic enmeshment. The difficulties that remained, however, suggest that there is something specific and irreducible in the experience of parents as a couple that enables an individual to sustain the full force of ambivalence and hostile feelings in an intimate relationship.

The clinical consequences of failure of the paternal function in psychic structuralisation, attended by a theme of real or threatened violence, have been examined in a number of significant contributions by British psychoanalysts. Fundamental to this has been the work of Glasser (1996) and his concept of the 'core complex', in which the consequences of failed individuation and the threat of engulfment by the primary object are encapsulated in the agonising dilemma of being able neither to sustain closeness with the object nor to survive apart from it. Glasser understood perverse sexuality as an erotised version of the raw, self-preservative violence aroused by terrors of engulfment. This permits the object to survive and relations to continue, but on the basis of sado-masochism, which, however subtle, is the essence of all perversion. A recurrent motif in the histories of his patients is that of the father who has failed to interpose himself and mediate the child's relations with a narcissistic mother. Such fathers may be absent and unavailable, but may equally be present but passive and disregarded (Glasser 1992).

Campbell (1995) identifies the task of the father in opening up the mother–infant dyad, as having two aspects: he must draw the mother back into adult sexuality and, at the same time, lay claim to his child in an independent relationship. He argues that suicidal enactment is based on a delusional fantasy of merging with an idealised mother through the destruction of the body and may be a consequence of an internalised father who has failed adequately to protect and hold his son in mind. Schachter (1999) offers further reflection in this area. Considering a disturbed woman's use of repeated abortion in an effort to free herself from her controlling mother, Pines (1994) refers to the image of an ill and disregarded father, with little power to protect his wife and daughter from their deadly entanglement. In Fonagy and Target's account (1999), the need for a father to support the child's development of a three-dimensional inner world of self-representation and reflection, becomes even more acute when a mother's difficulties prevent her from recognising and confirming her child's experience as separate from her own. In her account of the use of violence as a vehicle variously of autonomy and of fusion with the object, Perelberg (1999) focuses on the distorted fantasy of the primal scene, as it was conceived by a patient trapped in a desperate enmeshment with his narcissistic mother.

The patient

Mr R began three times weekly psychotherapy with me after consultation with a male colleague, to whom he had been referred by his GP. Mr R was a fresh-faced young man of medium height and stocky build, untidily dressed in expensive but slightly ill-fitting clothes. There was an engaging earnestness in his manner and, oddly, for all his embarrassment and anxiety, a sense of presence about him.

Mr R was 33 years old and had been married for two years. He had a prestigious and demanding post in the City and had avoided taking any extended leave until his wife persuaded him to take a holiday abroad. While they were away Mr R told his wife that he was afraid to return to work. Despite positive appraisals he felt almost constantly anxious that he was not up to the job. He feared that he might be homosexual: he had never had, or wanted, sexual contact with a man, but fantasised about homosexual sex. Although Mrs R must have been upset by this, she accepted that her husband was committed to their future together and suggested that he must seek help from their GP. She has remained supportive throughout his treatment.

In his consultations with my colleague, Mr R spoke of disturbances in his early childhood and confusions and disjunctions in his later upbringing. He felt these experiences were important, but did not know how to think about them. More immediately distressing were the violent and masochistic homosexual fantasies that began in adolescence and were now an established part of his inner world. He also spoke of sexual inhibition with his wife since their marriage. Although he was not aware of sexual feelings towards other men, he felt tormented by the thought that he was actually gay but too weak to face up to the reality of this. Another fear was that he could become an alcoholic like his father. He accepted my colleague's suggestion of analytic treatment, but thought his demanding job would preclude him from attending more than once a week. Mr R's experience of these preliminary consultations remained significant for him throughout his subsequent analysis, both as a first encounter with analytic understanding, and as a sense that there was another person, a man, available in the background to his relationship with me. Nevertheless, at various points in his eight years' analysis with me he insisted that the consultant had said treatment should not exceed six months.

History

Mr R's parents met at Oxbridge, were married soon after graduation and his elder brother was born the following year. When Mr R was born three years later, father was an alcoholic and actively violent to his wife. Over the next few years he was almost constantly drunk and unable to work and mother was sometimes driven to call the police. When Mr R was four, mother left her husband and took both boys to live with her parents, while she found work and established a home for herself and her sons. There were several moves between then and Mr R's beginning secondary school. Although unsure about how much he actually remembered of his early life, he had a few clear memories: one was of his father hurling a plate at his mother. Another was of father standing at the head of the stairs shouting, in a way that terrified Mr R even to remember. A third memory was of mother carrying him because he felt too weak to walk from the car to his grand-parents' house. He felt that he had been very close to his mother throughout his childhood and increasingly dependent on her as each change of school left him more timid and isolated.

Father was absent from the family for about two years, having broken down after his wife left him. When he reappeared, he was no longer drinking and had begun to establish himself in the profession that would bring him wealth and success. With mother's active agreement the boys regularly spent weekends with father. Even now Mr R felt torn and almost tormented about this arrangement. Although he defended his mother's decision he had found these visits very uncomfortable. He longed for father's lifestyle, wealth and status which included classic cars and an expensive house, but felt disloyal to mother for resenting her more humble situation. At the same time he felt afraid of father, whom he described as 'strange' and having 'an odd effect on people'. As he was growing up, Mr R spent many hours discussing father with his mother. He thought that he had been 'trying to find out what father was really like' – as if father remained alive and available in mother's mind and he was trying to make contact with him, in a way that was impossible with the man himself.

For a long time Mr R's memories of adolescence were vague and inaccessible. One important event was that father paid for him to leave home and board for his sixth form at father's old public school. It was during this time that what Mr R called 'the gay fantasies' were formed and the characters who featured in them were based around boys at the school. These fantasies had remained essentially unchanged until his analysis.

Mr R did better academically in his sixth form than he had done in his years at state school and secured a university place. However, he lamented the fact that he had not followed his parents and older brother to Oxbridge and father's disappointment about this. He told me, with some bitterness, that he had become a 'Hooray Henry' in his first term at university in a desperate attempt to be the son he felt his father wanted. After several months of drinking and socialising, Mr R thought he had 'collapsed' spending most of his time alone, reading junk fiction, unable either to work or ask for help. Having failed his first year exams, Mr R returned to live with his mother, who was now married to her second husband. Mr R felt that this marriage had made a huge and unexpected difference for him. His stepfather, who was a practical man, unlike his own father, helped him to find his first job. Mr R thought that this was the first time he became able to stand his ground with his father and resist the latter's nagging phone calls. Mr R felt that his twenties, when his mother was settled, was the most secure and optimistic time of his life. By the end of this period, Mr R was well established in his field of business and in his relationship with the woman who was shortly to become his wife. He was shocked when his mother told him that his stepfather was an alcoholic and becoming increasingly disturbed and abusive towards her. Eventually the couple were divorced and stepfather moved abroad.

Mr R saw the failure of his mother's second marriage and her ensuing dependence on him in the early years of his own marriage, as the beginning of the difficulties that eventually drove him to seek help. In the aftermath of her separation and divorce, he found himself unable to work, drinking too much and sliding into the same malaise that he had experienced at university. The 'gay fantasies' were once again prominent in his mind and he felt increasingly possessed and tormented by them.

Although Mr R was able to recount these events and their impact on him, it would take a great deal of work in analysis to disentangle his feelings of anger, disappointment and, at a deeper level, disillusionment towards his father and stepfather, as well as the buried, bitter reproach he felt towards his mother for having married two violent husbands. I was interested by Mr R's narrative and struck by the urgency of his concern to present a coherent account of himself and his life. It seemed to me that he was close to being overcome by the confusion of his contradictory identifications, as well as from a profound ambivalence towards each of his parents, particularly mother. I felt that Mr R had presented me with a desperate scissors and paste job, drawing on all the memories, stories, bits of hearsay and projections from others at his disposal, in order to construct a narrative the coherence of which he could identify with. We arranged to begin work on a three times weekly basis after the summer break.

The analysis

First phase

The first three years of treatment were dominated by Mr R's oscillation between grandiose, magical 'all-at-once' expectations and undermining of his real achievements with an abusive self-denigration. He complained of feeling helpless and of being torn between two hostile worlds. On one side, there was the exciting, macho culture of his City job, driven by competition and achievement, with its promise of validation as a potent male, together with the threat of failure and humiliation, which left him constantly on the edge of being overwhelmed and 'smashed to pieces'. On the other side, was his analysis, where understanding could moderate the overwhelming 'too muchness' of his emotions and make them at least temporarily manageable. There, however, the feeling of 'at oneness' that he sought with me made me appear dangerous and seductive, recreating in the transference his entangle-ment and identifications with his mother. Mr R tried strenuously to main-tain the separateness of these two worlds, keeping his treatment secret from colleagues, in the belief that they already viewed him as a weakling. He was furious that I did not provide late evening sessions to obviate risk of comment on his leaving early or arriving late.

Mr R was astonished to recognise the parallel I drew between this current state of affairs and his situation as a boy, torn between the deep bond with his mother and the exciting, but emotionally dangerous contact with his difficult father. He was elated by the hope of resolution that such insights seemed to offer. Session after session, however, he returned crestfallen, having in effect 'forgotten' the powerful formula that was to free him from his difficulties. Gradually, he recognised the excitement and elation he felt with each fresh insight, and referred to this as the 'eureka' experience. With shame he admitted that once he left the room, he could hold very little in mind of what went on in his sessions. As time went by, I began to feel trapped by a sense of the futility and waste of this and of Mr R's masochistic submission to the bullying culture at work. It seemed that we each, in turn, were to be thrust in the role of mother as father's abused victim.

This period ended unexpectedly in Mr R making several errors at work, which enabled him, with unexpected good sense, to negotiate his departure from the firm. He then asked for five sessions a week and found work in another firm with a more benign and orderly management structure. As he became more settled at work and in analysis, he began to talk more seriously about how afraid he felt about his mind: he reported that his train of thought frequently seemed to 'cut out', leaving him, in effect asking himself, 'Am I on the right bus?' Generally, he disguised the extent of this blanking out but it left him in constant dread of being exposed as unable to think. Talking of this reminded Mr R of his puberty and early adolescence when he had first become aware of disruptions in his capacity to think. This was a time when, in terror, he tried to halt his body's development by shaving off his pubic hair and attacking and hurting his body, on occasion, smearing himself with excrement. The intrusion of violent, sexual thoughts made thinking and studying impossible and made him afraid that he was going mad. He thought that his terror from this period had never fully receded, but had eased when he went to boarding school at 16.

After the subsequent summer break, I felt there was something more solid and 'put together' about Mr R as if his clothes fitted him better. For some weeks his material was dominated by his difficulties in managing a disruptive young woman who was a member of his team. When senior management decided over Mr R's head to sack her, he felt bitterly humiliated, but also terrified of her possible response: would she rubbish him as ineffectual or accuse him of her victimisation and make him feel guilty? Mr R said that he wished he had a 'real person' to talk to, but knew he would fall to pieces if he spoke of his helplessness outside of his sessions. I said that he could not bear me to be a real person who could think about him: I must either be 'at one' with him, with no mind of my own, or else – a familiar image – a computer giving him printouts on what to do. I suggested a parallel between the belittling 'not quite real' relationship with me, which he felt did not help him, and the tangled, destructive involvement at work, which belittled him but which part of him wanted to hold onto. Mr R did not disagree but was clearly annoyed. The sado-masochistic enactment in all of this became clearer next day, when I said that Mr R found it hard to know how powerful he felt his colleague to be. He told me that, for the first time in a session, he had a flash of the gay fantasies – as if to cut out what I was saying. He said that he probably was afraid to recognise that he might actually invite people to abuse and mistreat him. I said that that he felt badly treated by me recently and pushed to think of painful things. Mr R replied seriously: 'Yes, and if I'm doing that with you, who's on my side, how much more dangerous is it for me to look for ill treatment with people who are not?'

The reality of Mr R's dread of the couple and his imagined version of the primal scene now began to emerge. He came to a session worried about a change in the management structure at work, which he tried to explain in a confused and roundabout way. Eventually I said that I thought he was telling me that there were to be two distinct hierarchies, each led by a powerful individual and that he was answerable to both of them. Mr R agreed that this was so and that he was sure he would end up being shat upon. He was silent for several minutes, then said, 'I'm thinking about what I told you I used to do to myself.' The session ended there.

Next day Mr R was still shaken. He said that he thought he now had no option but to tell me about the 'gay fantasies'. Although he had referred to the fantasies before, what was happening now seemed different: as if in some formal way he was opening them up and surrendering them to the analytic work and to me. The fantasies were formed in his years at boarding school, his first extended separation from his mother. Each began with himself and one of several other boys from school, whom he identified as equally vulnerable and effeminate, embracing in a loving way. At a certain point, several very masculine boys would burst in and degrade them, forcing anal and oral sex on them simultaneously, finally leaving them both on the floor 'like a pile of shit'.

Mr R told me that he felt afraid of what he had begun. I said that I thought he felt afraid that I was robbing him of his fantasies and the power they had for him, and that he was terrified of feeling empty and helpless without them. Mr R agreed and then went on to describe the structure of the fantasies, which always used pairs of individuals disposed in intricate patterns and engaging in predetermined practices. Each pattern and practice had a code linked with a playing card, so that, in a remarkable interplay of passivity and control, the events of any fantasy were determined not by Mr R directly, but by chance and the draw of a card. As he found himself reflecting on the fantasies for the first time, he was amazed by how vivid his memories of boarding school were, in contrast to his muted sense of things in the present. He thought that this might have to do with his wanting to blank out the reality of his life in the here and now. He said he thought of himself as 'only half a man', as I thought silently about the 'half' people on playing cards who were stuck together, end to end. It was the end of the week and Mr R was apprehensive about how he would manage the weekend.

He arrived for his Monday session in a terrible state and I felt a wave of anxiety as he began to tell me about this. For the previous 24 hours he had felt possessed by a demon. He knew that this was in his mind but not in a controlled way, as his fantasies were. He felt as if he was being physically shaken and feared he was going mad. He had been so terrified that he had spoken to the local priest, who had said that what he described did not sound like demonic possession to him. He thought Mr R would be sensible to continue working with his analyst. Mr R said that he now feared that I would be furious with him or else hurt – because he had spoken to the priest. My anxiety had, in fact, subsided as I heard about the priest and his cooperative response. I said that Mr R. seemed absolutely desperate, as if he had been seized by something much bigger than himself which was going to shake him to pieces. At the same time, he was terrified of being trapped between two people who were meant to help him but who hated and wished to destroy one another. Mr R agreed with this and said he had imagined the priest and me saying bitter, critical things to each other. He paused and said he was thinking about his parents and his father's violence to his mother somehow it always seemed to come back to that. I agreed and said: 'Look, this has to be conjecture – but we know that a tiny child feels very close to its mother. The very physical experience that you brought today and the terror that went with it made me think that it was to do with you being very close to your mother identified with her really when she was being battered and terrorised by your father.' Mr R said he thought that there was some-thing in this. He was silent and then, in a strained voice, wondered about something he had never dared think before: had his father been sexually violent to his mother?

In the following sessions, Mr R was calmer, his thinking seemed firmer and I had a sense of something more lively and engaged in him. He told me that his father had rung to complain about something and that Mr R had been unusually firm with him. I made some comments based on my assumption that father was an overtly aggressive and bullying man. Mr R said that this was not the case in any obvious way: father was difficult to relate to because he was intensely manipulative, constantly complaining of being badly treated, in a way that got right inside. It made Mr R feel helpless and absolutely terrible and he knew that father had this effect on other people too, particularly his mother. He said his rows with father in the past had been due to father's manipulativeness. He now wondered why it was that he could stand up to his father once his mother had remarried. I said that perhaps he could take the risk because mother had a man to protect her and him. (I later thought that mother's husband might also place limits on Mr R and protect him from the extremes of his own murderousness.) Mr R said that this was probably right; he realised that he had never been able to think about father in this way before, although father had always been present in his mind and he had always felt burdened by him.

This sequence of sessions revealed for Mr R – and for the analysis – the powerful force connecting the violence between his parents in his early years and his current intense anxiety and shaming sexual fantasies. His dread of feeling overwhelmed and helpless beneath the fury of two warring forces had come alive in the session and he had believed it was about to be enacted in the transference by an analyst who would be hostile to her patient's need for a supportive second object. From our reconstruction – however speculative – of what might lie behind the powerful somatic force of Mr R's terror, we recognised that, on some profound level, Mr R felt totally identified with his mother and her experience of being battered and terrorised. This reconstruction offered Mr R an alternative to his sexually charged fantasies as a means of mastering and representing psychically this overwhelming, unprocessed experience. Although the task before us was substantial, he had now found a position from which to think about himself, his parents and his history in an active and constructive partnership with his analyst.

The force of Mr R's perverse, masochistic solution remained considerable, as did his concern to engage me in an enmeshed, over-solicitous enactment. When he returned from a business trip the following week, he reported feeling burdened and fearful. This struck a slightly false and self-dramatising note. I said that he needed to impress on me how awful he was feeling, otherwise he was afraid I would be out of touch and unavailable to him. Mr R conceded that his trip had gone well and that he had reason to feel satisfied with himself. He was silent for the rest of that session and at the start of the next. Eventually, he said that he felt strange: not 'upset' as he expected, but cut off and very low, as if everything around him was dead and he was at the bottom of a deep well. The session proceeded slowly, with long silences and heavy, opaque feelings. Mr R said that both his terror and distress of the previous week and the gay fantasies seemed very far away. I wondered if one purpose of his sexual fantasies was to distract and shield him from the sort of feelings he was having now. Mr R told me that he was thinking of a dark place like a well and that he had reached a kind of flat bottom and was smoothing himself out in his own mind. He felt as if his life was becoming continuous for the first time – all the events, family history and connections. Previously, he had felt that everything in his past was crumpled up, like a piece of paper, and that nothing in it made sense. We talked for a time about these two images of his life: crumpled, with no proper beginning or end and lacking connections between events and this new feeling of continuity, stretching back to the awful early years. He could now see things as taking place in time and over time, not in the 'all-at-once' way that was totally overwhelming. Mr R said that he thought that something very important had happened in this session. He sometimes referred to it in later years, regarding it as a crucial turning point in his analysis.

The sense of having a reflective distance between himself and his troubled history was new to Mr R, as was a capacity to recognise and think about his father's intrusiveness and manipulation. We had began to understand his masochistic fantasies as his 'own private theatre', a defensive structure against feelings of helplessness and confusion that he had contrived in adolescence in response to the demands of reality and Mr R's terror of his growing sexual body. With the hope of no longer feeling entirely identified with his parents' violent past in an overwhelming, 'all-at-once way', he began to sort out the differences between his father and himself and to untangle the confusions between his self-representations and the representations of father in his mind. He found himself listing qualities that he saw in father, qualities that were his own and qualities that they had in common. He also spoke sadly about wishing he had a 'proper father'. He remembered several men who had been supportive and available when he was a boy, including an admirer of mother whom, he now realised, he and his brother had wanted her to marry. Mr R knew that his father had had a difficult relationship with his own father and he feared that this unhappiness would pass down the generations. He had been relieved that his first child was a girl and was now hoping and fearing that the baby his wife was carrying would be a boy.

Mr R recognised his wish to get into a fused, 'at-one' relationship with me that continued, with various degrees of conflict, to be a central theme of his analysis. It now reminded him of the urgent, repetitive conversations that he had with mother about his father, particularly during his adolescence. He now thought that his struggle to get hold of a sense of father in his mother's mind had led him, paradoxically, not to separateness, but to becoming even more tangled up with her. Around this time I became aware of a shift in my counter-transference response to Mr R, from being almost too empathic and containing to sometimes quite impatient. On a couple of occasions, I caught myself cutting in prematurely, with an intrusive and unnecessary interpretation. Having thought about this, I said to Mr R that I believed that his sexual fantasies reflected his sense of being caught between his parents and filled up with their terrible destructive feelings, as well as with his own rage about his situation. In the excited, sexualised enactment of fantasies, it seemed that within the intimate confines of his private theatre, he cast himself as the victim of a violent, intrusive assault by two people, at both ends, as a means of transforming the terror and desperation of his mother's and his own experience.

In the following sessions, Mr R talked about his dread of thinking. He had begun to recognise how much energy he spent on keeping thoughts from his mind, for fear of the damage and destruction that would follow. Even now, he was often terrified that having a particular thought would immediately make it become real. He realised that he had desperately needed a father to give him a sense of boundary and the limitations of what is possible. His actual father was enigmatic and confusing: intrusive, manipulative and complaining when present, or else absent and unavailable. Beyond this, lodged somewhere in his own and/or his mother's memory, was a figure of explosive and crushing violence, whom it would be catastrophic to either identify with or oppose.

Mr R said it was difficult to let himself know what his father was like and how angry he felt towards him. I linked this anger with his attacks on himself and his own potency, both in the fantasies and in his professional life. He became upset and told me that there was something on his mind that terrified him: he had had a feeling of sexual arousal while playing with his daughter the previous week, when she leant against his genitals. I said that while the notion of abusing his daughter horrified him, it also served as a profound attack on his idea of himself as a father. Next day he said it was a relief to have voiced his fear, but he was now afraid that he might have disturbed my mind and put me in a panic. I took up his fear of how powerful and destructive his thoughts might be and his wish to lodge them in other people's minds – 'just as you felt your parents did to you'. Mr R said that for years he could not bear the thought that his perverse and violent fantasies had had anything to do with his father yet he had always known that this was so.

This period of work allowed us to identify Mr R's perverse fantasies as an attempt to organise and structure his chaotic inner world and to impose a limited, sexualised coherence on his feelings of discontinuity and helplessness. The pull towards a magic, all-at-once solution continued, but he now began to find pleasure in realistic achievement – for example, he found a new satisfaction in playing the piano. Previously he had wanted to play magnificently to 'blow people's minds' with his rendition of the music and was easily discouraged and frustrated that he could not play with the power he imagined. Now he began to find pleasure in the music that he could play and from the sense that he was achieving more from practice.

Second phase

Mr R's career and family life became more settled over the next two years. His second child was a boy and Mr R was surprised and moved by his strong and tender feelings for his son. In analysis, we struggled with his concern to protect himself from becoming overwhelmed or seduced by separating and compartmentalising the various sectors of his life and his thinking. Mr R tried to hold me in mind as a benign and reasonable person, but sometimes his transference image of me as Kaa, the deadly, soft-voiced python of the *Jungle Book*, broke through, revealing his terror of engulfment by a phallic mother, her power unmediated by any man. He countered this terror with the guilty, hostile fantasy of me as a woman he paid to be always at his disposal. The covert and sexualised denigration in this fantasy was unmistakable, but it was difficult for Mr R to acknowledge his aggression. Although he told me that that his masochistic fantasies were less extreme and sometimes heterosexual, a substantial part of his violence continued to be managed and maintained in this split-off 'private theatre'.

The role of Mr R's aggression in the breaches and discontinuities in his capacity to think emerged strikingly in a Monday session. He arrived anxious and fretful about two of his colleagues having worked together to complete a task over the weekend. He was bland, evasive and then irritated when I reminded him of his fears about being ganged up on and cruelly excluded when two people got together either at work or here in analysis. After a silence he said that he was thinking of his parents' marriage as having 'sheared off'. He thought that we might have spoken before of his fantasies as 'shearing off' thoughts in his mind. He spoke of an image of a wall with a crack in it that had been papered over and how this does not work because the paper can split open. He supposed that this would be the 'shearing off'. He had never considered what had happened with his parents in this way before.

Mr R was preoccupied with this idea the next day, emphasising that he had remembered the previous session. He now used the image of an earthquake that makes great fissures in the ground to describe his childhood experience of his parents' divorce: standing either side of a fissure, being pulled either way and 'falling into a shitty place, full of shitty feelings – rage and grievance and guilt – and lying'. He said for years his anger had made him feel too helpless to think about it. Now for the first time he blamed his parents. He thought that I had probably tried to talk to him before about his rage, but he had been unable to take it in.

Listening to Mr R, I realised that there was something new in the way that he was speaking about himself: as if he was talking as an adult who was able to think about and feel for the child that he once was, without having actually to be that child. I spoke of this impression and Mr R said he was reminded of a novel in which a man can see that a 12-year-old boy is in a terrible state, with divorced parents and a suicidal mother, but the boy himself cannot see it. He thought that, like the boy in the novel, he had needed someone else to recognise how bad it was. Something had fallen into place that allowed Mr R to discover a more separate and reflective position in relation to himself and his history.

We had spoken about the absence of a proper, safe and present father as a man with whom to identify and as a partner for his mother, who would protect Mr R from his intense involvement and identification with her. Mr R often talked about leaving home to go to boarding school. He knew this had been his father's doing, but now he found himself struggling against a recognition that his mother had also been involved: on that occasion his parents had together discussed his future in a constructive and cooperative way. Mr R was surprised by his hostility to the idea of his parents as a more creative couple. He recognised that his fears of being on the outside of a couple might arise from his jealousy and aggression. The image of mother as his father's terrified victim – and of me confined to my consulting room awaiting his visits – served to protect him from his aggression and the retribution of an oedipal father.

Claiming his aggression and his place in an oedipal constellation allowed Mr R to think more clearly, continuously and honestly. He said that the damage that he thought he had done to himself in the past and present was to do with his rage and hatred and the way he had lied to himself and others, both about the state he was in and his hatred towards his father. Reminding him of the crack in the wall that forces the paper to tear, I said that I thought he was now talking about the fissure that he had made in his own mind so that he did not have to know about his hatred and fear. Mr R asked me sharply if I was talking about the fantasies because he thought they were about having to lie to himself about his father, pretending that he had wanted to be like father – imitating him with flash cars and drinking at university. All the time he was scared that he was unable to become a man at all. I agreed, adding that for him to become a man meant becoming someone dangerous and terrifying, as his father had been. Yet not becoming a man meant remaining always tangled up with his victimised mother. Mr R felt intensely anxious and then, as his panic subsided, began to talk about his struggle with impossible feelings in his teens. He said that now he could see that 'this awful ball of sex and violence' had gone into his fantasies. He paused, and then quietly said, 'I think a part of me became mad, a sheared-off part, so that I didn't become all mad.'

Mr R had an early session next day. I forgot to unlock the outer door, which left him ringing the bell but unable to get in for several minutes. He was furious and berated me for most of the session. He fell quiet then said that he was thinking that I must be feeling awful. Nothing like this had happened before and he had over-reacted, yet it was amazing for him to be able to be angry at all – and neither of us was wiped out. As he got up to leave, he looked at the ceiling and smiled. 'It's still there.'

Third Phase

Mr R's intense involvement with his mother, especially during adolescence, was central to his difficulties and to the splintered, 'sheared-off' quality of his inner life. Relations between them now were generally warm and affectionate partly because he was directing more overtly hostile feelings towards his wife and partly because of some obscure idealisation of mother, which carried on in the transference.

This area came to the fore in the seventh year of Mr R's analysis. The 'gay fantasies' were now less central to Mr R's life. He had been drinking too much for a time, but had stopped recently, recognising this as an attack on his self-awareness. He could no longer ignore his negative feelings towards his analysis, which he considered shameful, but necessary to maintain his confidence and capacity in the rest of his life. By the same token, his thinking was more free and available and there was a sense of urgency and directness. Talking about his mother and her privileged early life, he was suddenly furious with the mess she had made of it: 'A few years after graduating, she was the battered wife of a drunken husband!' Immediately, he felt guilty and then angry, embroiled in an angry, hair-splitting exchange with me. Eventually this led to the thought that there was something odd and contradictory about his mother: sometimes she was strong and competent, sometimes vulnerable, confused and readily intimidated. Thinking of this made Mr R intensely anxious.

In the following weeks, Mr R struggled with his wish to flee from analysis – and his fear that I would assent to this. He felt furious that analysis had exposed his desperate reliance on me and the fact that, for the most part, he avoided being aware of this dependency. We returned to his use of me as a woman for whose services he paid, who was waiting and available for him in my consulting room and whose job it was 'to pick up and process the shit'. He could no longer deny the ugly denigration of this or the aggression and irritability that sometimes marked his relations with his family – in contrast with his friendliness and charm in less intimate connections. He spoke of his subtle misuse of both me and of his wife – 'in order', he said, 'to be who I want to be in the rest of my life' and of how much he lied by pretending to be appreciative when underneath he was filled with spite and resentment. This last reminded us that recently he had remembered a period when he was 10 or 11, when he had delighted in secret misbehaviour: stealing, smoking and bunking off from school. There had been a quality of perverse triumph in some this: he had not only lied and stolen from mother's purse, but had sometimes used the money to buy her presents.

An unmistakable element in this account of Mr R's relations with his analyst, his wife and, in the past, his mother is the fusion of hatred and denigration with intense feelings of need, which is the essence of a perverse attachment. His capacity to disguise and disavow the reality of his sadism (except in the arena of his fantasies) was revealed in his transference image of me as a prostitute, working far from his home and place of work. About this time Mr R came across a book of pornographic photographs of adolescent boys. He was alarmed to find himself aroused by these images and by a fantasy of buying the book to show his wife. As I took up the violence in this there was a new sense of tension between us. Mr R acknowledged that he had been determined, on one level, to remain ignorant of the aggression and cruelty of his fantasies and to hand responsibility for dealing with them over to me. He spoke bitterly of his anger that I had not done so and that he was no longer able to split off and confine his awareness of his perversion to the consulting room. The 'private theatre' of his fantasies no longer worked, he said, and he was now being forced to recognise that its images of sexual cruelty were an essential part of his thinking, not some unaccountable, alien intrusion.

Mr R raged at having to maintain an awareness of his perverse ideation, as well as his dependence on analysis. He tried to confine this knowledge to a limited sector of his mind once again and, when this failed, threatened to end his analysis at the coming break. The deadlock was broken unexpectedly, when Mr R remembered a remark by the widowed mother of a friend to the effect that she had sent her son to boarding school 'because it wasn't right for a mother to be alone with her son'. As he spoke of this, Mr R was reminded of one of the pornographic pictures in the book: an adolescent boy being fellated by an older woman. This, in turn, made him think of his over-involved, over-excited closeness with mother in his early teens. Mr R spoke of feeling helpless, with his mind either 'blown' or 'about to blow' for most of that time. He was shocked, but relieved to hear himself say that he and mother had been 'caught up in something together' that was 'dangerous and terrifying', and that he had only got clear because his father had arranged for him to go away to school.

I reminded Mr R of the familiar experience in analysis, when some particular insight could rouse him to a pitch of excitement and sense of 'all-at-once' release ('eureka!') – only to end in collapse and hopelessness at the end of the session. He acknowledged this need to feel 'huge' with excitement: he had believed that this was the only way that he could amount to anything and be substantial enough to finish his analysis. As we thought about the intense, sado-masochistic, sexualised 'conversations' to which Mr R had clung over the years, he began to imagine a different sort of relationship. He asked me if I kept notes on his analysis saying that he hoped I did, so that there would be an account that was separate from what he remembered. I pointed to the contrast between this and several outbursts that had earlier revealed his hatred of my knowing anything independently of him. Mr R agreed and said that what was different was that he could now see beyond what had always been 'the conundrum' of our relationship: which of us was the stronger and which would be left helpless and disabled at the time of separation?

Confronting his need for an intense, orgiastic involvement with a key figure, inevitably enacted in the transference, allowed Mr R to think more freely and feel less ashamed of being in treatment. He was surprised that the people he told about his analysis were not shocked or horrified. He realised that the shock he expected was to do with his guilt and shame about the hapless dependency on his relationship with me and his covert vindictiveness and denigration of it. He noticed himself feeling more detached from his mother and able consciously to have critical thoughts about her. I had been struck by Mr R's vehement repudiation of the thought that mother might have played a part in the alcoholic collapse of both her husbands, as well as in his own difficulties. I suggested that, on some level, Mr R believed that his mother could read his thoughts and therefore his aggression towards her had been oblique and secretive, often acted out against himself. Mr R accepted this and was shocked to realise that the closeness between them had as much to do with her wishes as with his. He thought that the involvement had become particularly intense in his early teens, when he was in a desperate state, and that it had been the 'worst thing' for him. Previously, he had believed that 'hearing father's voice in his head' was the 'worst thing', but now he thought that perhaps I was right when I suggested that imagining his father's voice may have been an effort to protect and distance himself from mother.

This brought Mr R back to the way his enmeshed relationship with mother had 'come live' in his analysis in the 'eureka!' excitement of insights that he could not hold on to and that left him frustrated and furious. Now he recognised that I had been aware of, and had tried to speak to him about, what was happening between us. On the one hand, he had felt trapped and helpless in the relationship, and, on the other, angry that he needed my independent mind to help him understand something. Mr R was reminded of an image of Michelangelo's unfinished 'Captives': monumental figures that remain frozen in time, as they strain to free themselves from the enclosing marble. 'It's as if I've been trying to free myself from myself all this time.'

Mr R did not end his analysis at the break. There was still substantial work to do, but it seemed that we had finally established a sense of distance and space for reflection between us, as if there were now indeed a reliable father mediating our relationship.

Conclusion

Mr R, whose struggles I have described, was not directly the victim of his father's violence, which was directed exclusively at mother in the first four years of Mr R's life, before the marriage ended. He was unable to know how much his sense of an explosive penetration and assault was an independent memory and how much it came from an identification with his mother's experience, either at the time or through her later descriptions of this. In either event, Mr R's capacity for helpful, structuralising internalisation was compromised on various, crucial levels. He saw his father as someone damaged and damaging, impossible to identify with as a sexual male, particularly as adolescence approached, and on a much more fundamental level, we found that his inner, psychic space had long been penetrated by an awareness of the violence between his parents, which was almost somatic in its intensity. Defensive anality was manifest in all the complaints that brought Mr R to treatment: inhibition of purpose and creativity, thinking that was broken and discontinuous and a sense of being dominated by the demands of his 'private theatre' of (sado)masochistic fantasy.

Target and Fonagy (2002) argue that traumatising experience of, and with, the object in early childhood remains lodged within the self, blocking the elaboration of self and object representations, which provide for the triangulation on which an inner sense of space and temporality depend. In a distinct, but complementary formulation, Shengold (1988, 1989) describes the terror of annihilation and the upsurge of murderous primitive affect that is the consequence of primitive trauma, together with massive intensification of anal defensiveness that offer a bulwark against feelings of being overwhelmed. Mr R had maintained his precarious psychic balance since adolescence by compulsive use of masochistic fantasy. By this means he was able fleetingly to control and bind his identifications with a violent couple, which threatened to overwhelm and drive him mad. Mr R's perverse enactments and use of his body served both to erotise and to disavow the reality of his own violence and to support his denial of the oedipal order (Chasseguet-Smirgel 1984). His masochistic sexuality maintained his feelings of a privileged engagement with mother, which both threatened and excited him, while covertly reinforcing a sense of infantile omnipotence (Novick & Novick 1991). In all of this, Mr R was caught in the toils of an anal narcissistic universe of magic, all-at-once possibility and its opposite, despair (Grunberger 1979). The task of psychic structuring and the integration of disavowed reality, as well as of a healthy and effective aggression, was necessarily laborious, in time and over time, as is the nature of analytic work and inevitably incomplete.

References

Britton, R. (1989) 'The missing link: parental sexuality in the Oedipus Complex' in *The Oedipus Complex Today*, J. Steiner (ed.), London: Karnac

Burgner, M. (1985) 'The oedipal experience: effects on development of the absent father', *International Journal of Psychoanalysis* 66: 311–19

Campbell, D. (1995) 'The role of the father in a pre-suicide state', *International Journal of Psychoanalysis* 76(2): 315–23

Chasseguet-Smirgel, J. (1984) *Creativity and Perversion*, London: Free Association Books

Fonagy, P. and Target, M. (1999) 'Understanding the violent patient: the use of the body and the role of the father' in *Understanding Violence and Suicide*, R. Perelberg (ed.), London and New York: Routledge

Freud, S. (1916–17) 'The development of the libido and the sexual organisations', Introductory Lectures, *Standard Edition 16*, London: Hogarth Press

—— (1923) 'The ego and the id', *Standard Edition 19*, London: Hogarth Press

Gaddini, E. (1992) 'Formation of the father in the primal scene' in *A Psychoanalytic Theory of Infantile Experience*, London: Routledge

Glasser, M. (1992) 'Problems in the psychoanalysis of certain narcissistic disorders', *International Journal of Psychoanalysis* 73: 493–502

—— (1996) 'Aggression and sadism in the perversions' in *Sexual Deviation*, 3rd edn, I. Rosen (ed.), Oxford: Oxford University Press

Greenspan, S. (1982) 'The second other', in *Father and Child: Developmental and Clinical Perspectives*, S. Cath, A. Gurwitt and J. Ross (eds), Boston: Little Brown

Grunberger, B. (1979) *Narcissism: Psychoanalytic Essays*, New York: International Universities Press

Lacan, J. (1964) *The Four Fundamental Concepts of Psychoanalysis*, New York: Norton

Laplanche, J. and Pontalis, J.B. (1973) *The Language of Psychoanalysis*, New York: Hogarth Press

Lebovici, S. (1982) 'The origins and development of the Oedipus Complex', *International Journal of Psychoanalysis* 63: 201–15

Leowald, H.W. (1951) 'Ego and reality' in *Papers on Psychoanalysis*, New Haven, CT and London: Yale University Press

McDougall, J. (1989) 'The dead father', *International Journal of Psychoanalysis* 70: 205–20

Novick, J. and Novick, K. (1991) 'Some comments on masochism and the delusion of omnipotence from a developmental perspective', *Journal of the American Psychoanalytic Association* 39: 307–31

Perelberg, R. (1999) 'A core phantasy in violence' in *Psychoanalytic Understanding of Violence and Suicide*, London and New York: Routledge

Pines, D. (1994) *A Woman's Unconscious Use of her Body*, London: Yale University Press

Schachter, J. (1999) 'The paradox of suicide: issues of identity and separateness' in *Psychoanalytic Understanding of Violence and Suicide*, R. Perelberg (ed.), London and New York: Routledge

Shengold, L. (1988) *Halo in the Sky*, New York: The Guilford Press

—— (1989) *Soul Murder: The Effects of Childhood Abuse and Deprivation*, London: Yale University Press

Target, M. and Fonagy, P. (2002) 'Fathers in modern psychoanalysis and in society: the role of the father and child development' in *The Importance of Fathers: A Psychoanalytic Re-Evaluation*, J. Trowell and A. Etchegoyen (eds), Hove: Brunner-Routledge

Chapter 6

The problem of certain psychic realities: aggression and violence as perverse solutions[1]

Stanley Ruszczynski

Introduction

Both Freud and Klein understood psychological development as grounded in the interweaving of love and hate, life and death instincts, involving both the body and the mind. In health, in the context of a benign parental environment, the normal development of the infant's instincts results in the strengthening of the life instincts and hence the lessening in the power of destructive impulses. The aggressive element of hate is contained and comes under the influence of the capacity for concern for the other and therefore of love. Aggression may then be recruited in the service of passion and creativity and thus contribute towards the possibility of healthy relationships. As a result, true intimacy, which requires both the recognition of and respect for a separate other, becomes possible (Ruszczynski & Fisher 1995). Sex and, in particular, intercourse are experienced as reparative and potentially creative, arousing little or no guilt.

However, this benign integration of physical sex and love is one of the most difficult achievements of human beings' psychic development. The full expression of intimacy, love and sexuality requires the involvement of another, and this dependence on another, an affront to narcissism and omnipotence, carries with it the inevitability of feelings of ambivalence towards that other. The achievement of this capacity for ambivalence, in reality a lifelong struggle, is one crucial indicator of the potential for relatively healthy and mature relationships.

In the absence of this achievement of the capacity for ambivalence, love and concern do not temper and moderate aggressive instincts and aggression retains ascendancy. Fonagy has stressed the developmental need for

---

1 Parts of this paper were previously published as 'States of mind in perversion and violence' in *The Journal of the British Association of Psychotherapists* 41(2), July 2003. This chapter to be published in 2006 in *Clinical Lectures in Delinquency, Perversion and Violence*, S. Ruszczynski and D. Morgan (eds), London: Karnac.

normal aggression to be contained and writes that 'violence is unlearned not learned'. He says:

> [M]odels of aggression have tended to focus on how human aggression is *acquired*. Yet aggression appears to be there as a problem from early childhood, arguably from toddlerhood and perhaps from birth. Violence ultimately signals the *failure of normal developmental processes to deal with something that occurs naturally*.
>
> (Fonagy 2003: 190, emphasis added)

In such circumstances, relationships, sexual and non-sexual, are recruited in the service of malignant aggression and sexuality in particular may be hijacked and become expressed as sado-masochistic, perverse and destructive. Robert Stoller refers to perversion as 'the erotic form of hatred'. He writes:

> Think of the perversions with which you are familiar: necrophilia, fetishism, rape, sex murder, sadism, masochism, voyeurism, paedophilia – and many more. In each is found – in gross form or hidden, but essential in the fantasy – hostility, revenge, triumph and a dehumanised object. Before even scratching the surface, we can see that someone harming someone else is a main feature in most of these conditions.
>
> (Stoller 1977: 9)

Perversion

This understanding of the interlacing of sex and aggression, of love and hate, whether for loving or for malignant purposes involves both the body and the mind. It originates from Freud's delineation of mankind's 'Oedipal destiny' (Hartocollis 2001). Freud describes a 3- to 5-year-old boy's sexual attraction to his mother and his rivalry with and hatred of his father. He soon came to realise, however, that the young child pursues the love of the *opposite* sex parent with ambivalence because such a pursuit is feared to be at the expense of an affectionate attachment to the *same* sex parent. This dilemma is at the heart of the true nature of the triangular oedipal situation and hence feelings of ambivalence inevitably accompany any feelings of attachment, love or sexual expression.

Our oedipal destiny is the inheritance of these conflicting libidinal and aggressive wishes, residing within the psyche from the beginning of life. Those who followed Freud, and especially those within the Kleinian tradition, postulate that the triangular oedipal constellation is, in fact, confronted by infants from birth, because infants relate to their primary objects from birth, albeit in primitive ways. As such, libidinal and aggressive wishes are initially experienced in more absolute, narcissistic, fragmented and persecutory or idealised ways, inherent in the immature mind of the young infant, well before the classical Oedipus Complex is reached.

Britton has elaborated an additional dimension to the oedipal situation by highlighting that, as well as relating to the parents individually as mother and father, the young child, driven by natural curiosity, is confronted by the dim realisation of a special link between the two parents, namely their sexual relationship (Britton 1989). Children have to come to tolerate not only their exclusion from that special parental relationship, but also that the parental intercourse has a special quality because it may lead to the creation of a baby. Here is a highly charged and psychically demanding attack on the infant's omnipotence and narcissism.

The working through of the various elements of the oedipal situation is parallel to what Kleinian writers refer to as the psychological development from the paranoid-schizoid to the depressive position. These positions refer to constellations of anxieties and defences that create particular states of mind and object relationships, the former more primitive and based on processes of splitting and projective identification and the latter resting more on a recognition of and concern for a valued and separate other.

To make this monumental developmental move the child has to come to tolerate what Money-Kyrle refers to as the irreducibility of certain 'facts of life', which have to be accommodated to, among which he includes dependence and the supreme creativity of parental intercourse (Money-Kyrle 1971). Similarly, Chasseguet-Smirgel has described the need to come to terms with 'the basic elements of human reality: the double difference between the sexes and the generations' (Chasseguet-Smirgel 1985). She has suggested that failure to do so results in a regression to an 'anal universe', where separateness and difference is disavowed. Segal too suggests 'the building of a "faecal empire"' as a defence against separation (Segal 1972). The language used by these writers, 'human reality', 'facts of life' and references to the defensive reassertion of anality, suggests the fundamental necessity of coming to tolerate the anxieties and hatred caused by this loss of narcissism and omnipotence when confronted with difference and separateness.

Developmental difficulties might emerge at the threshold between the more primitive, narcissistic states of mind and the more mature depressive position. At this borderland, libidinal and aggressive instincts and hence the expression of love and hate, life and death forces, come into problematic conflict. If the loss of narcissism and omnipotence feels intolerable, if the capacity for ambivalence cannot be achieved, if hate retains an ascendancy over love, then aggression, violence and the disavowal or perversion of painful realities are likely to emerge as predominant expressions of emotional states.

Freud initially understood perversions as residues of infantile component drives that had not been sublimated. In his 'Three essays on sexuality', Freud (1905) describes as perverse the regular intrusion into the adult's sexual life of the normal polymorphously perverse sexual and aggressive instincts of childhood. These partial instincts make up aspects of the ordinary and appropriate sexuality of children; some such behaviour may be contained in adult fantasies and in the foreplay of some peoples' ordinary sexual lives. What significantly differentiates such activity from a perversion is that perverse activity is compulsive, fixed, driven by hatred not love for the object and does not usually culminate in heterosexual inter-course leading to orgasm.

Although it is tempting to think that sexual perversions are primarily sexual and driven by sexuality, they are better understood as activities that *hijack* sexuality (Caper 1999), recruiting it to accomplish ends that are fundamentally aggressive and destructive, resulting in what Stoller calls 'eroticised hatred'. The subject or patient himself is also a victim of this violence and hostility, certainly in his mind and sometimes in his physical body, although this will often be overshadowed by the fate of his victim.

A significant development took place in Freud's understanding of per-version when he recognised the significant defensive functions of perversion, defending primarily against knowledge of aspects of the Oedipus Complex (Freud 1919, 1927). We would now say that what is perverted is knowledge of reality, both internal and external. This hatred of and attack on reality is likely to be a product of both the narcissistic and omnipotent aspects of the patient's personality and a defensive reaction to the unbearableness of the pain, humiliation and subsequent murderousness likely to have been experienced in their upbringing. The successful disavowal of reality requires sadistic control of the object and a splitting of the ego, creating an uncon-scious object relationship based on control and misrepresentation. Hence such relating is primarily sado-masochistic, perverse and based on cor-ruption of truth. In working clinically with perverse and violent patients, couples and individuals, I have come to find it useful to hold in mind the idea of *violation* as a central element in the sado-masochistic and violent act. It is essential to think not only about disturbed and disturbing violent or perverse behaviour, but also about a *perverse organisation of the mind*, based on a particular constellation of anxieties, defences and internal object relations, which will get projected into the external world in a variety of ways (Ruszczynski 2003). The violent act violates the other's body and their mind; the sexually perverse act is also likely to violate the other's body but the overriding central dynamic in the perverse act is the corruption of the other's mind by corrupting truth and reality albeit often by sexual and aggressive means. I will say more about this later.

The core complex

Glasser (1979, 1998) holds the view that central to the understanding of a perverse psychic structure is a dynamic psychic organisation, which he calls 'the core complex', in which aggression is an integral feature. The core complex has two elements and is a normal phase of development through which the infant has to pass. It describes the constant movement between the deep-seated longing for the most intimate closeness with the object, usually understood to be the mother – closeness to the degree of merger or union – and then a terrified flight away from this object because the desired merger threatens to result in the annihilation of the self.

Glasser goes on to suggest that this threat of annihilation may be dealt with in either of two ways. One way is a defensive narcissistic withdrawal. This is likely, however, to produce a sense of desolate isolation and abandonment, leaving only the self (both body and mind) as the focus for the aggression initially directed at the object. This may lead to a profound level of depression. Alternatively, the threat of annihilation by the engulfing object may provoke intense self-preservative aggression, acted out or in the mind, which, while aimed at securing the survival of the self, involves the destruction of the object, usually considered to be mother. Often, it is this aggression, if acted out, that brings the patient to the attention of the authorities or alerts the patient themselves to the dangerousness of their phantasies and impulses.

Both the narcissistic withdrawal and the aggressive attack on the primary object produce, in phantasy, the loss of the desired object and the terror of abandonment. This propels the patient back towards a desperate search for closeness and merger with the object and fear of engulfment may then re-emerge. Here we have the psychically disturbing circular nature of the core complex.

Henri Rey (1994) describes a similar psychic structure when he refers to the 'claustro-agoraphobic' dilemma, which leaves the patient feeling that a place of safety and security cannot be found. Closeness to the desired object results in feelings of intrusion and claustrophobia, separateness from the object results in feelings of abandonment and agoraphobia. Similarly, Lewin and Schulz (1992) refer to the core pathology of the borderline patient as the 'double danger of losing or fusing'.

Such anxieties about engulfment and abandonment arise from the more infantile and primitive aspects of the personality, which appear to dominate the adult mind. We are referring, therefore, to an underlying psychotic structure with narcissistic and omnipotent features and a preponderance of primitive or psychotic anxieties, defences and object relations. Intrusion into and mastery over the object is more likely than a capacity for concern or intimacy. Corruption of reality to meet narcissistically driven needs is equally more likely than a toleration of dependence, separateness, loss and ambivalence.

Faced with these overwhelming primitive anxieties, an attempt might be made to defend against them by *sexualisation*: the defensive manoeuvres of narcissistic withdrawal or self-preservative aggression become eroticised.

This sexualisation defends against the anxiety of the loss of the self or the other by creating the phantasy that, rather than engulfment or abandonment, there is an interpersonal object relationship.

The sexualisation of aggression results in masochism or sadism. When there has been a narcissistic withdrawal, only the self is available to receive the aggression initially directed at the threatening object. When this aggression directed at the self is sexualised, it leads to masochism. The masochist has a sense of control over the degree of suffering that will take place; there may also be a phantasy of control over the threatened abandonment and the feared annihilation. In addition, the masochist may feel that he is clearly not being aggressive to the object, who is therefore safe from his destructiveness. Unconsciously, the masochist also experiences the suffering as punishment, allaying some of the guilt for the aggression felt towards the object:

A masochist man, who uses a dominatrix to torture and humiliate him, some time into treatment, is beginning to let himself know of his terrifying sense of emptiness, loneliness and resultant feeling of unworthiness. The pain and punishment he receives from the dominatrix temporarily relieves him of these feelings because with her he is the architect, not the victim, of his suffering and humiliation. By eroticising the pain and abuse he gains pleasure from the experience as well as from the fact that he now has ultimate control over what is done to him. He behaves in a highly dangerous manner so as to omnipotently defy humiliation, suffering and terror, living out a phantasy that he can not only control but also ultimately survive and overcome the abusing hateful internal object, whose victim he felt himself to be. This is all in the service of gaining some sense of triumph and mastery over otherwise unbearable feelings and fantasies. This particular patient is also unconsciously punishing himself for having failed to rescue his mother from her depression and pain.

The sexualising of self-preservative aggression, by the same token, results in sadism, a wish to hurt and to control. In phantasy, this preserves the object, which is now no longer threatened with destruction but is engaged with, albeit sadistically. It is not unusual to see this in couple relationships where one or both partners treat the other with hatred and contempt but cannot separate.

The sexualisation, masochistic or sadistic, acts like a binding force, organising and securing the object relationship. Sadistic and masochistic relating are ways of engaging intensively with an other so as to militate against the dangers of separateness, loss, loneliness, hurt and destruction. Excited, intense feelings and experiences are used as substitutes for love and care. The excited eroticised repetition serves to defend against destructiveness, both one's own or that of the other. There is pretence that it is a kind of loving relatedness, an exciting exchange sought by both parties.

The differentiation between self-preservative aggression and sado-masochism is important in understanding the difference between the object-relating of the perverse patient and the violent patient. The differentiating factor is the attitude to the object at the time at which the act is carried out (Glasser 1979, 1998). In the *self-preservative aggressive* act, the destruction of the object is essential and its purpose is to eliminate the other who is perceived as life threatening. The object's emotional reaction, the meaning of the behaviour to the object, is irrelevant. The violent act is, in phantasy, life preserving. It seeks psychic equilibrium. This is a violent and cruel state of mind and, at the extreme, is murderous. The *sadistic* act, contrariwise, seeks to torment and control the feared other whose emotional reaction is crucial: the specific aim is to cause the object to suffer, physically or mentally. As sado-masochism is based on this control and domination of the other, it requires *some*, albeit primitive, capacity to imagine the other's state of mind.

These states that I have described are, of course, never as clear cut in reality. Domination and control are essential features in both aggression and sadism. In self-preservative aggression, they are sought only to negate the danger while in sadism they play a central role in entrapping and engaging the object. Let me give two clinical vignettes as illustrations:

> A young female patient was referred for depression but also because she often found herself in disturbing sado-masochistic relationships. She had been raped on at least three separate occasions during her adolescence and early adult life. As a child she had been abused, emotionally and physically, first by her father and then, after being taken into care, by two sets of foster parents. She presented as generous and self-effacing, willing to put herself out for anyone, friend, neighbour or stranger. Her masochism, however, was barely hidden behind this pseudo-caretaker role and as treatment started it soon became clear how she ignored obvious signals of danger, often placing herself in positions where she could be manipulated, abused or raped. She often missed sessions and complained that I was not offering her times that she could manage. In the transference, I became the inconsiderate and uncaring object and she the suffering victim. When she did attend, she would often say that it was for my benefit and not hers. Her partner abused her emotionally and, in effect, raped her for his sexual satisfaction. She masochistically sustained their relationship in the face of obviously cruel and violent treatment and triumphantly told me how she was prepared to survive his abusive behaviour because, she said, she had never felt as loved by anyone as she did by him. In the clinical

work, we came to see that in this masochism there was, in phantasy, a secret triumph over hurt, neglect and abuse. But to sustain this illusion of control and domination over her situation, she had to deceive herself about the degree of abuse she suffered. She corrupted the reality of being used and abused into a fantasy of 'being loved'. Occasionally, this perverse structure broke down and she became physically ill. Briefly, she would then feel murderous fury at her partner who continued to pay her no attention and persisted in demanding that she meet his requirements. Unconsciously terrified that her murderousness would destroy her object, she would rapidly reconstruct the masochism and re-establish her benign view of the relationship and, in the process, split off and evacuate her own feared aggression. To do otherwise would require her to face the pain and rage at the multiple losses, betrayals and abuses that she had experienced and that fundamentally threatened her sense of psychic and bodily survival. In the transference, I became the abusing object seen as 'forcing her' to think about her internal world and the ways in which she dealt with it.

A homosexual paedophile patient, who used young homosexual male prostitutes, started off his contact with a new prostitute in a mutually consensual sado-masochistic relationship, with him taking the overtly masochistic role. Initially, he believed that this encounter would turn into a mutually loving relationship and that this might eventually help the prostitute to develop a better life, a manic and omnipotent idea that revealed the primitive nature of his thinking. When the prostitute inevitably let him down, my patient began to fear losing him. Initially, his masochism increased, often at great personal cost, psychical and financial, in an attempt to secure the relationship. When this inevitably failed to secure the continued interest of the prostitute, my patient found himself having extremely sadistic and violent fantasies. It was his anxiety about acting on these fantasies, together with a growing sense of oscillating between this sense of murderousness and suicidal despair, which eventually led him to seek treatment.

As is implicit in both these brief clinical vignettes, *there is always deception involved in masochism* – a secret contempt and desire to control is hidden behind the appearance of humiliation and submission. *Beneath masochism there is always an unconscious phantasy of omnipotent mastery over the feared and hated object and the masochistic sexualisation of the fear and hatred results in perceived pleasurable gratification from the suffering.* A masochist is therefore *always* at the same time, a sadist, even though either the active or passive aspect may be the more strongly developed and represent the predominant activity.

The facts of life

Since sado-masochism is understood to be such a central feature of all perverse activities, we are led to the conclusion that there is always deception, misrepresentation and an attack on reality in the perverse act. And, because the perverse mental structure involves the whole personality, *the attack on or misrepresentation of reality is a fundamental and central feature of the perverse patient's psychic makeup*:

> A female patient, multiply abused and violated in her childhood and adolescence, who now gets herself sexually abused by picking up men in the street and parks or sex clubs, said to me recently, 'I can't stop doing this because I would then have to know what I was doing.' She often refers to herself by a different name when she describes her very dangerous and perverse activities and says that she does not know this person who engages in these frightening masochistic behaviours.

Clinical perversion may therefore be understood as fundamentally defensive, achieved primarily by deception and disavowal of reality, with the purpose of fending off unbearable affects that would otherwise have to be known and experienced. Perverse phenomena could be described as deriving from destructive forces directed primarily against perception, both the perceiving self and the other who might prompt these perceptions. Perverse patients might therefore be described as unconsciously determined to pervert the capacities for thought and perception, not only their own but also those of people around them, including, of course, clinicians and other carers (Feldman 2000).

A number of writers have paid particular attention to the understanding of perversion as the product of distortion and misrepresentation of reality. They stress, in particular, the disavowal of the reality of *the difference between the sexes and between the generations* (Chasseguet-Smirgel 1981, 1985; McDougall 1972; Steiner 1993). For example, the paedophile denies the reality of the differences between adults and children and, in doing so, denies one of the fundamental facts of life, that of the difference between generations. The transvestite may need to diminish or obliterate the reality of the difference between male and female:

> One transvestite patient describes how successfully, in his view, he divides his life between his male self and his female presentation. When cross-dressed, he thinks of himself as a woman and acts out various scenarios as if, in his perception, he is a woman. When not cross-dressed he leads an ordinary life as a man: he is married with children, has a sexual relationship with his wife and is professionally successful. He considers himself to have complete mastery over whether he is a

man or a woman. He can be both, he says, with whichever gender role he is dressed up in being the gender that he considers himself to be. Although he talks of the differences between the two genders, we have begun to understand that actually he denies that any differences really exist. In his mind, the differences are spurious or marginal – really there are no differences and he can transcend what there are at will. What is emerging in the clinical work is the view that there is a gulf between the genders such that each constitutes a separate universe, which cannot possibly be bridged. This seems to imply a very disturbed image of the internal couple – a fused and undifferentiated couple or a couple who are completely unknowable to each other. Either way, there seems little possibility of the couple relating to each other. This has rather pessimistic therapeutic implications for the possibility of this patient even beginning to integrate the different aspects of himself in a more realistic way.

Misrepresentation of reality is central to an understanding of the perversions and arises from a specific mechanism in which contradictory versions of reality are allowed to coexist simultaneously. Freud initiated this understanding of the coexistence of competing realities, in his study of fetishism (Freud 1927), but the mechanism described is applicable more broadly (Steiner 1993). Freud says that the young boy assumes that there is no difference between the sexes. After the child is confronted with his observations of the reality of the differences between the genders, he may accommodate his powerful assumption of no difference by simultaneously holding the belief that his mother *does* have a penis while retaining his knowledge that she *does not*. The fetish is a substitute for the mother's penis that the little boy believed she had, a belief he does not want to give up, even when faced with material reality, because it raises castration anxieties: his anxiety that he too might suffer a similar fate and lose his penis. This holding on to contradictory beliefs is achieved by what Freud calls, 'a rift in the ego, which never heals but increases as time goes on. The two contrary reactions to the conflict persist as a centre-point of a splitting of the ego' (Freud 1940: 276). Chasseguet-Smirgel suggests that this splitting be considered as a vertical split in the ego, with the perverse disavowal of reality existing *alongside* the recognition of reality (Chasseguet-Smirgel 1985).

Money-Kyrle's delineation of three fundamental facts of life may be helpful to further our understanding of this perverse relationship to reality (Steiner 1993). These are: 'the recognition of the breast as a supremely good object, the recognition of the parents' intercourse as a supremely creative act, and the recognition of the inevitability of time and ultimately death' (Money-Kyrle 1971: 443).

The first fact, that the source of goodness required for the infant's initial survival comes from outside him (usually from mother), challenges omnipotence and narcissism and requires the toleration of separateness, dependence and gratitude. In the paranoid-schizoid position, mechanisms of splitting and projective identification make possible illusions of omnipotence and narcissistic self-sufficiency. In the course of development, there begins to be some integration of this omnipotent wish for self-sufficiency with the painful realisation of attachment and dependence. However, this realisation of separateness and dependence might feel too threatening and a defensive perverse structure may be created to accommodate a partial acceptance of the reality of separateness, difference and dependence but coexisting with a continued belief in omnipotence and self-sufficiency, with the latter retaining a primacy.

Aspects of this disavowal of separateness and dependence are often part of the psychic structure of abusive and violent marriages. In such marriages, there appears to be a relationship between two separate people, but actually one or usually both partners are relating narcissistically, whereby, as a result of projective identification, the other person is actually seen as little more than an extension of the self. This is a perverse relationship because the partner's separateness is disavowed and they are, in effect, colonised and related to parasitically. When this colonisation is felt to be challenged by the partners' ordinary independent behaviour, it might feel very threatening to the narcissist because it requires a toleration of separateness and dependence and hence a loss of omnipotence and narcissism. If this is felt to be intolerable, violent reactions might follow that are both an expression of the threat to the narcissistic self and a means of trying to recapture and control the other. Aggression and sado-masochism emerge as ways of dealing with the reaction to, and fear of, separateness and dependence.

The second fundamental fact of life described by Money-Kyrle is that of the true reality of the oedipal situation. This involves, first, tolerating knowledge of the parents' sexual relationship and tolerating being excluded from it; second, tolerating the generational differences between adults and children; and, third, recognising the differences between the sexes, which includes coming to know that babies come from heterosexual intercourse.

The reality of these facts of life can be denied by the solutions offered by some of the sexual perversions: these can be thought of as attacks on separateness, difference and the procreativity of the parental couple that cannot be tolerated. For example, the difference between the generations is denied in paedophilia and child sexual abuse. Homosexual intercourse might be understood in the clinical situation as an attempt to deny the differences between the sexes and to deny that new life is the product of the intercourse of these two sexes. Transvestism might be thought of as an attack on sexual difference:

> A transvestite patient states with total conviction that, when cross-dressed, he believes himself to be a woman. He recently described the

very specific way in which he holds his penis when masturbating thereby simulating, he thinks, a woman masturbating using her clitoris. When cross-dressed he straps his genitals in such a manner that they are, in effect, forced back into his body, demonstrating his abhorrence of his penis and his attempt to eradicate the reality of its existence.

The third of Money-Kyrle's facts of life relates to the realities of passing time, of loss in its multiple forms and ultimately death. Facing and mourning losses, a constant necessity throughout life, is part of the reality of life that may feel so unbearable that loss is disavowed. This is connected with the pain of recognising that from the beginning of life all good things have to come to an end, starting with the fact that access to the breast cannot go on for ever. This makes us aware of the reality of its existence in the external world outside of our control (Steiner 1993) and is an affront to any notions of our omnipotence and narcissism.

Sohn has suggested that some extremely dangerous and violent patients may be understood partially in relation to their experience of loss. He describes how their condition may be the result of a developmental history punctuated by a profound series of losses and a failure in the development of the capacity for symbolisation (Sohn 1997: 72). For such patients 'loss has been totally and psychotically denied' resulting in a psychological condition, 'in which total intolerance for any depressive experience leads to a need to act out physically' (Sohn 1997: 70). Hyatt-Williams too suggests that a state of murderousness is derived from a failure to work through emotional disturbances engendered by experiences, thoughts, feelings and phantasies to do with loss, life-threatening situations and death (Hyatt-Williams 1995):

> I am reminded of one patient who was often preoccupied by cruel and murderous fantasies, especially when stimulated by news reports of brutal attacks, sexual abuse, killings or other such horrors. He was regularly involved in physically aggressive and violent encounters in his relationships and with near strangers, believing that this was the only way he could manage himself, his experiences and other people.
>
> He began to be confronted by a sense of loss and endings, as a result of our addressing the beginnings and endings of sessions, holidays and other breaks in the treatment, transitions in the therapeutic relationship that he found almost intolerable. Initially, he oscillated between despair and rage at me: he said that I had 'invented' time and forced him to realise that he was neither omnipotent nor immortal, that time does pass on, that things do come to an end and that he cannot control any of it. His fragile and defensive narcissism had previously allowed for an illusory sense of timelessness and a phantasy of immortality so that losses need never be confronted and mourned. When he could not

avoid awareness of loss he found himself getting involved in physical fights, often coming out the loser but feeling in some way cleansed by the experience. In addition, throughout his adult life he had had a serious of completely unnecessary facial cosmetic operations in the attempt to maintain his perceived youthful appearance. When we eventually discussed this, his terror at the idea of loss, including the loss of his own youth through the natural process of aging, was experienced as if a life and death matter. The loss of his youth was closely attached to an idea of him having 'blemishes', which in his mind explained why he had been consistently rejected, abused and discarded in his child-hood. This impossibly persecuting standard of perfection was also applied to his objects and came to be understood as a desperate defence against the extremely imperfect objects who had deserted him (his father died when he was one) and abused him (his mother emotionally and his aunt and subsequent carers sexually). Later in the treatment, when the reality of loss, including the passing of time and ageing began to be more tolerable, he became shocked by his propensity for violence and by the medical assault he had perpetrated on himself. We slowly came to see that he had turned to both sadistic and masochistic aggression and violence to sustain a sense of triumph over the unac-ceptable losses and ravages of time and the physical and emotional blemishes that this inevitably produced. This had also helped him fend off the murderous hatred of his imperfect objects who, in their attitude and behaviour towards him, had defined him as imperfect, to be discarded or abused.

Perhaps in a less dramatic way, promiscuity might be one sexualised attempt to deny the passing of time when a constant seeking of new sexual conquests is used as a false reassurance to counter the realities of passing time, of ageing and its attendant losses, ultimately death. Resorting to the timelessness of fantasy, be it romantic or base, might be another way to deny and overcome this fact of life. The narcissism and omnipotence that is severely threatened by this psychic reality might be further bolstered through phantasies of timelessness and immortality It is only with the acceptance of time passing that time itself becomes a factor in patients' lives. Losses may then become more tolerable.

In his paper on fetishism, Freud (1927) refers to two patients both of whom were unable to face the loss of their fathers through their premature death:

> I am reminded of a late adolescent patient, referred for assessment and treatment following an indecent exposure and other sexual offences. He told me that he had talked to his father about the incidents which he now felt he understood. I knew, as did he, that his father had left him

and his mother about 14 years previously, when the patient was about 3 years old, and that he had not seen him since. Given that he had this relationship with his father, the patient told me, there really was no reason to discuss the offences with me, especially as his father completely understood him, as I obviously did not.

Another patient, who had violent fantasies about capturing, torturing and mutilating women talked at some length, in his assessment, about his relationship with his father. It was only when I, in passing, made some reference to his contact with his father that the patient then told me that his father had died nearly 30 years ago when he was 6 years old.

Both of these patients found themselves having sadistic fantasies towards women and the first patient was beginning to enact these. Both spoke of profound difficulties in their current sexual relationships and described women as desired but also profoundly feared and experienced as intrusive and overwhelming.

Glasser has written that, 'what offers a different solution to those found by the pervert and the psychotic is . . . the presence of the father. With the father present, the infant can seek a solution to the core complex's "irreconcilable conflict of opposites" by turning to the father as an alternative object' (Glasser 1985: 409).

I wonder whether the inability of these two patients to tolerate and accept their father's death prevented both of them from successfully completing the mourning process. It was as if each felt their father to be present although they both also knew, because they were not psychotic, that he was actually long absent or dead. Had they been able to tolerate their losses and mourn, they may have been able to integrate the father as an internal figure. He could then have been made use of intrapsychically as required when managing the core complex oscillation between abandonment and annihilation in relation to the mother.

Violence and sadism as perverse solutions

Perverse beliefs, sado-masochism and violence are turned to defensively when ordinary psychological development inevitably moves the patient towards having to recognise, tolerate and integrate these facts of dependence, oedipal realities and the inevitability of loss. If these psychic realities are felt to be unbearable, perverse activities are enacted and perverse beliefs are developed to both suppress the knowledge of these realities and also to corrupt the mind's capacities to perceive and tolerate them. Simultaneously, the disavowal of certain facts of life, for example the significance of generational differences, legitimises some sexual perversions and acts of violence. Denial and aggression are turned directly against the mind of the patient and through projective processes against the mind of his or her objects. Developmentally this locates such patients at the border of the paranoid-schizoid level of functioning.

Some patients act out perverse solutions in grossly perverse or violent acts. Others do not, but their states of mind and object relationships will be heavily influenced by perverse solutions. There appears to be no agreement as to the difference between those patients who actually act out their phantasies and those who do not, but it is very probable that destructiveness in the character is crucial in the perverse personality. Whether this excessive destructiveness is constitutional or whether it be the result of parental and/or environmental deprivation is open to debate and discussion. Probably both are present.

The crucial difference between those patients who actually act out their violence and perversion and those who do not might be related to a failure in infantile containment (Bion 1962). This would lead to a failure in the capacity to achieve some depressive position functioning and a failure in the capacity for symbolisation (Sohn 1997). Some patients turn their perverse solutions into fantasies or dreams, but others have no capacity for such mentalisation and so have to act them out.

Hyatt-Williams and Sohn, among others, have suggested that enactments of aggression, violence and murderousness are induced by the psychic toxicity resulting from certain emotional experiences being unprocessed as a result of a failure or lack of containment (Hyatt-Williams 1998; Sohn 1997). Fonagy and Target (1995) assert that violence is a product of the person's lack of a capacity for reflection or mentalisation. Without the experience of containment, no development of a psychological self can take place, a self that can process and think about experiences and psychic states. This cannot happen because such development requires the primary experience and perception of oneself, in another person's mind, as thinking and feeling. Fonagy and his colleagues make this point powerfully when they write that: 'Freud, arguably, saw infancy as a time when the self saw others as extensions of itself . . . our emphasis is the reverse – we see the self as originally an extension of experience of the other' (Fonagy, Gergely, Jurist, & Target 2002: 8). Without this experience, the sense of self is rooted, not in the mind, but in the *body*. The incapacity to psychologically reflect on and integrate mental experiences results in the person having only the body and bodily experiences through which to provide a sense of relief, release or consolidation. Borderline, perverse and violent patients often speak of a profound sense of relief and peace following an act of violence or a suicide attempt.

The lack of a containing function leaves persecutory and toxic object relationships festering in the mind, constituting a cruel and threatening presence that has to be annihilated for self-preservation. The capacity to deal with this psychologically is non-existent or extremely fragile. It can only be dealt with physically, using the body. If projected, it may result in a sadistic, violent or murderous attack on the body of the victim. If identified with it becomes masochistic or results in a suicidal attack on the physical self.

In thinking about failure in containment and the resulting sado-masochistic and violent interactions, we should probably also keep in mind the nature of the death instinct, which, at its strongest, attacks and distorts the capacities for perception and judgement, both in the potentially available containing object and in the self. It is a useful construct if it is thought of as a destructive *psychological* force (Feldman 2000; Segal 1993). What is deadly about the death instinct is the way in which meaning, and specifically difference, is attacked, resulting in the retardation of the development of a thinking psychological self (Feldman 2000) and hence creating what Chasseguet-Smirgel calls the perverse patient's 'substitute reality' (reported in Leigh 1998).

Conclusion

We might say that our oedipal destiny obliges us to manage, tolerate and find creative expression for our aggressive and loving feelings in relation to the realities of life, especially those of dependence, the double difference between the sexes and the generations and the inevitability of loss. This involves giving up narcissism and omnipotence, recognising our dependence on others and tolerating loss, all of which require us to contain the inevitable feelings of ambivalence, of love and hate, separateness, difference and gratitude. If this can be achieved, the interlacing of sex and aggression becomes available for expression in the service of creativity and passion in whatever arenas of life and relationships.

If, however, the lack or failure of containment, resulting in an incapacity for mentalisation, combined with the strength of the death instinct, does not allow for the toleration of these fundamental facts of life, the aggression aroused recruits sexuality and becomes acted out, defensively, in sado-masochistic, perverse or violent ways. The interlacing of sex and aggression is then recruited in the service of the hostile disavowal of the facts of life and is destructive of the realities of life and of the creative potential of relationships.

References

Bion, W. (1962) 'A theory of thinking', *International Journal of Psychoanalysis* 43: 306–10
Britton, R. (1989) 'The missing link: parental sexuality in the Oedipus Complex' in *The Oedipus Complex Today*, London: Karnac
Caper, R. (1999) *A Mind of One's Own*, London and New York: Routledge

Chasseguet-Smirgel, J. (1981) 'Loss of reality in the perversions – with special reference to fetishism', *Journal of the American Psychoanalytic Association* 29: 511–34

—— (1985) *Creativity and Perversion*, London: Free Association Books

Feldman, M. (2000) 'Some views on the manifestation of the death instinct in clinical work', *International Journal of Psychoanalysis* 81: 53–65

Fonagy, P. (2003) 'Towards a developmental understanding of violence', *British Journal of Psychiatry* 183: 190–2

Fonagy, P. and Target, M. (1995) 'Understanding the violent patient: the use of the body and the role of the father', *International Journal of Psychoanalysis* 76: 487–501

Fonagy, P., Gergely, G., Jurist, E.L. and Target, M. (2002) *Affect Regulation, Mentalisation and the Development of the Self*, New York: The Other Press

Freud, S. (1905) 'Three essays on sexuality', *Standard Edition 7*, London: Hogarth Press

—— (1919) 'A child is being beaten', *Standard Edition 17*, London: Hogarth Press

—— (1927) 'Fetishism', *Standard Edition 21*, London: Hogarth Press

—— (1940) 'Splitting of the ego in the process of defence', *Standard Edition 23*, London: Hogarth Press

Glasser, M. (1979) 'Some aspects of the role of aggression in the perversions' in *Sexual Deviation*, I. Rosen (ed.), Oxford, New York, Toronto: Oxford University Press

—— (1985) '"The weak spot" – some observations on male homosexuality', *International Journal of Psychoanalysis* 66: 405–14

—— (1998) 'On violence: a preliminary communication', *International Journal of Psychoanalysis* 79: 887–902

Hartocollis, P. (2001) *Mankind's Oedipal Destiny*, Madison, CT: International Universities Press

Hyatt-Williams, A. (1995) 'Murderousness in relation to psychotic breakdown (madness)' in *Psychosis – Understanding and Treatment*, J. Ellwood (ed.), London and Bristol, PA: Jessica Kingsley

—— (1998) *Cruelty, Violence and Murder*, London: Jason Aronson

Leigh, R. (1998) 'Panel reports: perversion', *International Journal of Psychoanalysis* 79: 1217–20

Lewin, R.A. and Schulz, C. (1992) *Losing and Fusing: Borderline Transitional Object and Self Relationships*, Northvale, NJ and London: Jason Aronson

McDougall, J. (1972) 'Primal scene and sexual perversion', *International Journal of Psychoanalysis* 53: 371–84

Money-Kyrle, R. (1971) 'The aim of psychoanalysis' in *The Collected Papers of Roger Money-Kyrle*, D. Meltzer and E. O'Shaughnessy (eds), Strath Tay: Clunie Press

Rey, H. (1994) *Universals of Psychoanalysis in the Treatment of Psychotic and Borderline States*, London: Free Association Books

Ruszczynski, S. and Fisher, J. (1995) *Intrusiveness and Intimacy in the Couple Relationship*, London: Karnac

Ruszczynski, S. (2003) 'States of mind in perversion and violence', *Journal of the British Association of Psychotherapists* 41(2): 87–100

Segal, H. (1972) 'A delusional system as a defence against the re-emergence of a catastrophic situation', *International Journal of Psychoanalysis* 53: 393–401

—— (1993) 'On the clinical usefulness of the concept of the death instinct', *International Journal of Psychoanalysis* 74: 55–61

Sohn, L. (1997) 'Unprovoked assaults: making sense of apparently random violence' in *Reason and Passion: A Celebration of the Work of Hanna Segal*, D. Bell (ed.), London: Duckworth

Steiner, J. (1993) *Psychic Retreats*, London and New York: Routledge

Stoller, R. (1977) *Perversion: The Erotic Form of Hatred*, Sussex: Harvester Press Limited

Part III

Destructiveness in disguise and as disguise

Misanthropy and the broken mirror of narcissism: hatred in the narcissistic personality[1]

David Mann

> It fills me with depression – reduces me to utter despair to see men living as they do. I meet with nothing but base flattery, injustice, selfishness, treachery, villainy everywhere. I can bear it no longer. It infuriates me. I mean to fling my gauntlet in the face of the whole human race! . . . I hate all mankind, some because they are wicked and perverse, others because they tolerate wickedness – because they don't show the unrelenting detestation that virtue owes to vice.
>
> (Molière, *The Misanthrope*, Act 1)

The occasional state of temporarily hating everybody or permanently hating a section of the population is so common we could probably consider both to be within the 'ordinary' range of human feelings. Indeed, recent research (Hess 2000) suggests that the average person usually has at least three others he or she hates at any one time. We might say that our love, if not for humanity as a whole, extends at least to some sections of the population or individuals and this keeps any global hatred in perspective: we recognise exceptions and distinctions; we recognise the difference between those we love and hate. We could say that, in this ordinary way, love offsets hatred. Misanthropy is a psychological state distinct from this in which mankind in general is permanently hated. Misanthropy is a pathological position whereby all people are hated: love is conspicuous by its absence.

I will begin by first describing some of the general features of misanthropy and its relationship to narcissism. This will be followed by a clinical example followed by further discussion.

In misanthropy, the hatred of mankind extends to the self, there are no exceptions so the misanthrope can only hate himself as well. However, a distinction is usually to be made between self and other. The misanthrope

---

1 An extended version of this paper was published in *Love and Hate: Psychoanalytic Perspectives*, D. Mann (ed.), Brunner-Routledge (2002).

considers he or she has an insight into the human condition, knows the truth that others are blind to and, therefore, is placed in a position different from the rest of humanity. In that respect he or she is special. This is the essence of the narcissistic component of misanthropy.

To the misanthrope, humanity is hated for its ordinariness. The very ordinariness of humanity is experienced as gross acts of violence against the narcissistic self. Small acts of lack of consideration are exaggerated and given inflated levels of importance in the psyche. Human achievements in art, science, law, culture or civilisation are either ignored or denigrated as false disguises to the true brutality underneath. All virtues are considered insincere, concealing the iniquities inside.

At the heart of this hatred are instinctual, animal and bodily characteristics. All behaviours and psychologies associated with aggression, sex, eating, defecation, disease, ageing and other bodily functions are hated and resented. The phrase 'I hate your guts!' succinctly highlights the body-based nature of this hatred. The misanthropic ideal would be a disembodied mind, free from the body and bodily desire. Misanthropes are inclined to experience others as 'crap' or 'shit', or the world as a sewer – thereby identifying humanity as nothing more than a defecatory function or product. Humanity is not seen as a beast with a brain but just as a beast. Curiously, the beastly nature of the animal kingdom is denied. Offset with the hatred of humanity is an idealisation of nature, a non-human world free from the polluting and corrupting influence of people. The animal nature of animals is acceptable precisely because it is not filtered through the prism of human desires. Essentially what is hated is all human desire and need for others. It follows that the ultimate ideal is of a peopleless world where the misanthrope can live in harmony by him- or herself, alone with nature. Love, if it exists anywhere, resides only in the non-human environment. But love is the wrong term here: strictly speaking it is more a question of non-hate, nature is not loved but idealised because of the absence of the hated human race.

This narcissistic fantasy is also the source of the deepest narcissistic wounds: misanthropes hate people and wish to do away with them, yet at the same time are forced into confronting the limits of their own destructive desire: humanity can be destroyed only in fantasy. Misanthropes stand powerless, like King Lear cursing into an indifferent storm, a storm that pays no attention to their hate. Kernberg describes the deepest layer of the narcissistic relationship with external objects as the source of the misanthrope's pathological defences. 'It is the image of a hungry, enraged, empty self, full of impotent anger at being frustrated, and fearful of a world which seems as hateful and revengeful as the patient himself' (1974: 219).

Despite the misanthrope's destructive desires, humanity continues to survive. Winnicott (1971) has described how infants need to be able to destroy their parents in fantasy while at the same time needing the parents to survive their annihilatory hate: this will help infants to get a sense of the limits of their destructive fantasy and also confirms that whatever their wishes, the parents can still survive. With the misanthrope, a different process operates: the survival of the object does not put the fantasy into a realistic perspective. On the contrary, the rage is intensified through frustration and impotence; the object's survival is experienced as a narcissistic wound that adds further fuel to the hatred.

Generally, the narcissistic dilemma is that the person wishes to be free from the need for others; ideally, the narcissist would like to be entirely self-sufficient. The problem from the point of view of the narcissistic fantasy is that such an individual is highly dependent on others. This need for others, especially the need to be at the centre of the other's desire, is what grieves narcissistic personalities, faced as they continually are with the obvious and mortifying proof that they are not the most important person in the world.

This process of dependence and hatred of dependence on others is found in misanthropic thinking and perpetuates the misanthrope's loathing of mankind. Misanthropes see themselves as different from all the rest, in fantasy wishing the population to die, yet confronted with the failure of their wish which is both mortifying and wounding. Both Kohut (1966) and Ledermann (1987) emphasise the narcissist's inability to love others. I consider this is partly an attempt to define narcissism by what is lacking rather than by what is present. Narcissistic personalities are not really indifferent to others, even if they claim to care about nobody. In fact, that is part of the narcissistic problem: they can never be free of an attachment of sorts to others. We can define narcissism as an absence of love for objects but it is probably more accurate to say that it is rather a surfeit of hate that overwhelms and floods all the relationships. Narcissism is more accurately described as a pathological disorder of hate.

The misanthrope is a particularly extreme form of the narcissistic hateful attachment to the object. Hate binds the misanthrope to humanity in general and everybody in particular, including the self that is despised for its impotence and bodily functions shared with everybody else. The narcissist's body unites them with everybody else and therefore denies them separateness and unique specialness. Neither can the misanthrope seek sanctuary as a hermit. They remain persecuted not only by the knowledge that humanity exists all around them but also because they are persecuted from within, the hatred turning against the self for all that it holds in common with everybody else and for the failure to reap the benefits of annihilatory fantasies. There is no love anywhere, either inside for the self or for others outside. The hatred is maintained by being caught in a self-perpetuating circuit of hating humanity for its animal ordinariness (that is to say, the presence of human desire), seeing the self as different and special because the misanthrope 'knows' the truth but yet the misanthrope's body and the need for recognition as special can only lead to self-hate because their body unites them and their specialness is not recognised by others. This narcissistic wound fuels the hate so the cycle continues: humanity is hated afresh with renewed vigour, only resulting in renewed narcissistic wounds.

We can think of extreme narcissistic hate as a defence against unbearable loss, abandonment or disconnection from others. Although striving for uniqueness, the narcissist's grandiosity results in a proliferation of connections to others where, in fact, none ordinarily exists. Hatred thus unites and binds the narcissist to every available object no matter how inconsequential it is in reality. This is a passionate connection that defends against separateness. The absence of connection is experienced as unbearable discontinuity of being. There is no capacity to be alone in Winnicott's (1958) terms. Separateness would equal annihilation, a fall into an abyss, an emptiness, a wilderness, a solitary confinement of infinite magnitude. Hatred, by expanding connections, maintains a relationship to the entire human race.

Developmentally, the world that is hated is that of the mother. Possibly because the mother was too frustrating or unavailable or projectively identifying her own unconscious hatred into the baby, the infant is left bitterly disillusioned in the goodness of life. Instead there is a retreat into an anal universe (Chasseguet-Smirgel 1984; Mann 1997: 162–79) where all differences are intolerable. Hatred is thus both an attempt to control the mother and compel her into satisfying the infant and also allows the infant to avoid the painful feelings of disconnection and abandonment. Ultimately, such hatred is a defence against narcissistic wounding.

If we consider narcissism as a disorder of inordinate and excessive hate, or as the domination of hate in the psyche, we can examine the myth of Narcissus afresh. Narcissus was exceptionally beautiful but heartlessly rejected his lovers. His lovers must have felt lust rather than love as there was nothing about his personality that was appealing, 'for he had a stubborn pride in his own beauty' (Graves 1955: 286): clearly a handsome but odious brat! His relations to other are hateful and sadistic, Echo is scorned, and his most insistent lover, Ameinius, is given a sword by Narcissus to kill himself with. Ameninius commits suicide with the sword but invokes the gods to avenge his death. The god Artemis hears the plea and exacts the vengeance by causing Narcissus to fall in love with himself. When Narcissus kills himself it is with hateful despair and grief that he cannot keep his reflected image. Hate thus is more prominent than love throughout the myth. The myth might also shed some light on the origins of pathological narcissism.

I have refrained from entering the debate about whether narcissism is a primary or secondary phenomenon resulting from parental failure. The myth seems to suggest a mixture of constitutional factors, primary narcissism, since Narcissus is born exceptionally beautiful (suggesting constitutional factors), but also parental intervention: trouble befalls Narcissus once the god Artemis (parent figure) intervenes (suggesting secondary processes). This suggests to me that narcissistic personality disorders are a mixture of constitutional factors that may or may not become problematic depending on parental intervention. With less than good-enough parenting the infant's narcissistic disposition may suffer the severe wounds that lead to the difficulties of the narcissistic personality.

In ordinary circumstances hatred is not totally self-consuming. Indeed, hate may have many developmental advantages. Gabbard (1993) sees hate as helping to maintain a separate sense of self experienced from the disappointments in the other. The ambivalence in oedipal renunciation means all subsequent relationships must have a degree of hatred. Therefore, hate is developmentally inevitable as the child's demands will clash with those of the parents. Ordinarily, objects of our hate remain split off or isolated from other areas of our life so hate does not corrupt all our relationships. The misanthrope's problem is that there is nothing in opposition to hate that can attempt to modify or balance its phantastical power.

Other writers have seen positive aspects to hate. For example, Kernberg (1993) has seen hate as a core affect 'which contributes to the formation of the aggressive drive'. Kernberg (1995) describes how hate requires sufficient ego development to allow differentiation between self and object representations. Unlike Freud, he recognised lesser degrees of hate that do not necessarily wish to destroy the object, for example, a wish to humiliate or make the object suffer.

Blum (1997) points out that turning away from the purely destructive aims of hate requires the capacity for self and object love. Therefore, it requires the ego to differentiate self from other. With these capacities the ego can tame and neutralize aggression and severe and persistent hate are less likely. Hate is developmentally normal and can be used as a motivating force. It is normal to hate our enemies or those that torment others. He also notes that hate is readily elicited by narcissistic injury and easily intensified through identification with hated or hating objects. It would therefore be of interest to explore whether hate is always an aspect of narcissism or whether hate exists independently of narcissistic issues. Freud's (1918, 1921) comment on hate arising from the 'narcissism of minor difference' (I would add there is plenty of hate arising from large differences too) seems to suggest that hate is generally associated with some narcissistic wound.

Hatred, then, has a place, alongside love, as part of the ordinary experiences of passion. Generally, hate serves positive narcissistic functions contributing to the individual's capacity to make distinctions between what is good and bad for the self and those we love. It is also worth reminding ourselves that, as Kohut (1966) demonstrates, narcissism is not necessarily pathological but contains positive functions in normal psychological development. Normal narcissism gives us a healthy enjoyment of our own activities and successes and helps us adapt to disappointment and anger at our own shortcomings and failures. Kohut suggests that healthy narcissism is an essential ingredient in all creative activity. However, the narcissistic personality seems to get none of the benefits either from normal hate or normal narcissism. Their hate is too consuming and too inclusive. The problem for the misanthrope is that hate becomes attached to the narcissistic component of the personality and, through grandiosity, takes on a greater significance. In the absence of any capacity to love or the ability to be indifferent, the hate has no restrictions or boundaries and thus becomes the sole source of relationship to self and others. Misanthropes do not experience their relationships as creative. Even when they achieve a superficial appearance of goodness or love, their underlying unconscious relationship is one of hateful destructiveness. Their hate disables their functioning so that all their – external and internal – relationships become hateful. They can feel special, different from the rest, even superior to all humanity, but their sense of uniqueness is not about possessing or giving something life enhancing to others: rather, their grandiose uniqueness keeps them isolated from others. The hate results from the terrible disappointments and the rage this induces makes contact with others or themselves too painful.

What I have been trying to describe in the misanthrope's mind is the pathological pervasiveness of hate that dominates the total psyche in the absence, and without the mitigating influence, of love. Pathological hate and ordinary hate have a different relationship in the psyche. The ordinary mind contains a plurality of competing passions of differing, but usually unequal, strengths. Ordinary hate has its place in the psyche alongside other affects and passions: one feeling, albeit a particularly powerful one, among many. The misanthropic mind contains no plurality of affects and passions, rather a totalitarian dictatorship of hate. In this narcissistic pathological hate there is nothing else.

In a world of total hate, how can something good, like love, exist? This is the crux of the therapeutic problem posed when the misanthrope seeks psychotherapy.

Clinical material

Jonathan came seeking psychotherapy for his long-standing depression. He had a history of alcohol and stimulant abuse, although when I began seeing him he had used neither for four years. He had given up alcohol after waking one morning and not recognising the woman in bed next to him; he was deeply shocked when he eventually realised she was the woman he had been living with for 10 years. During the period of his intoxicated lifestyle he led a violent life. At one point he was considered for inclusion in an armed robbery, but, on reflection, the violent gang he was associated with dropped him as he was too unstable and unpredictable. His own description of that part of his life was: 'I was an animal in the 1980s, a thug.' Although he was no longer violent he could still be verbally abusive, his favourite phrase being: 'Why don't you eat shit and die?!', that is to say, a projection of himself as full of shit. He was aware that a lot of people were frightened of him.

He made his misanthropy clear from our first session where he defined one of his therapeutic goals as: 'It would help if I could just hate people without them knowing it. My hate of people drips off me: they know it in seconds.' This was followed by instant hate about anything I might have to offer. My initial enquires about his childhood and relationship with his parents brought the retort: 'Don't give me any of that fucking Freudian crap,' which I took to mean he wasn't interested in my thoughts. He did say, though, 'I was breast fed on vitriol,' but offered no further comment.

Slowly, over the next few months, he did give a picture of his childhood. He thought his past was 'full of shit' but there would be nothing left if he got rid of it, he was now 'just full of crap with my head stuck up my arse'. Father was an alcoholic whose drinking frequently left the family in poverty. He was described as extremely violent to everyone: 'It was blood on the walls kind of violence.' Jonathan also saw another side: his father was a skilled craftsman but his low self-esteem left him too embarrassed by his occupation to want to involve him or pass on his craft. Although his relationship with dad was bad, he felt he had some understanding and compassion for where his father was coming from. Not so for his mother. She was described in the vilest terms, she would get him and his brother to compete against each other for money: 'Great mothering skills, fucking ragbag shit cunt!' He thought she was attractive on the outside but a 'dirty, smelly bitch otherwise'. He added, 'I can understand why my dad wanted to fuck her, but why did he want to breed with her?!' He thought his mother turned him against all women who he saw as a 'foul, stinking mess but good to fuck now and then'. This was not straightforward misogyny, though, in a way his hate for mother was projected out by turning the whole world into her. His father was also hated but perhaps less so than his mother.

His hatred for his parents spilled out onto the rest of the world. He expected people to undermine him; sometimes he felt everybody was better than him or else they were all shit; he hated the world because he hated himself so much. His mother had said she thought he considered himself better than everybody else, he replied he was. He said he would not feel lonely if a nuclear bomb wiped out the human race. He thought people were crap, although when I queried this he conceded there were decent people about. He felt he was like a satanic king, a Midas, except that everything he touched 'turned to shit not gold'. 'I'd make a fucking good dictator,' he said after a particularly bad week. He tried to live life mostly as a hermit but because his hatred was for himself and his internalised parents, solitary confinement brought limited relief as he remained persecuted by his internal world of objects.

A good deal of his therapy was filled with his disgust at himself and others. He commented that, unlike most people, I did not seem frightened of him. Indeed, I was not, in fact, I knew I quite liked him. He was never overtly aggressive with me or threatening. However much he hated the world he was clearly trying to preserve something better with me. His hatred of therapy would be expressed in other ways: he frequently missed sessions when he felt too bad to leave his house. He was very repetitious in his material which was often presented in a joky, self-depreciating manner and he frequently said how little he trusted me. At this time I considered my attitude to him to be essentially positive, but I was aware I was coming to feel increasingly bored in the sessions. I would become alert only when notable new material was mentioned or his colourful use of swearing delivered a memorable phrase. His sessions were filled with long periods of tedium punctuated with scraps of material that would suddenly excite my interest. I did not realise the extent of my counter-transference until after a summer break when I reviewed the previous year's work by looking over my clinical notes. I noticed that my entries were getting shorter, they often began with the sentence 'Same sort of stuff' followed by a brief elaboration but one entry described the whole session in a single word: 'Usual.' I was reducing all his sessions to sameness in the same way he treated the human race: dehumanised, devoid of individuality and treated as a faecal mess with no nutritional value. I suddenly recalled his early therapeutic goal of wishing to hate people without their knowing it. In effect, I had been hating him without knowing it, although perhaps he had detected it. I was hating his thoughts because, as he told me in the first session, he hated my Freudian thoughts. His misanthropy was contagious. My boredom had been an expression of my hate for him. I was shocked at this revelation, although I then came to realise that perhaps the situation was not quite so bad. I knew I still had warm and positive feelings for him but, whereas before I assumed that that was all, now I was aware of just how ambivalent I had become with the emergence of more negative hateful feelings.

Having come to some understanding and acceptance of my own hate that left the small matter of trying to do something useful and less destructive with it. I confronted him more about his hateful attacks on the therapy but whereas I had underestimated my hate, I had overestimated his. He said that, apart from occasionally thinking I was 'a smug bastard', which was quite a compliment by his usual standards, he trusted me more than most people as he knew I was trying not to harm him. That genuinely confused his stereotype of people. Over the next few months he had more confusing experiences. He was given a lift by a genuinely nice family who had a disabled child, they had no reason except natural generosity and kindness to do him a favour. He had felt so overwhelmed in their car that he had to get out early. On another occasion he reported spending 10 minutes with his parents that were unexpectedly pleasant and rancour free. He became more real and trusting in therapy and eventually began to tell me of his sexual abuse as a child from his older brother and sister and later from a paedophile. I had suspected something of the kind but he had rebuffed my initial enquires during his assessment with 'I wouldn't tell you if I had'. More importantly, his long-standing relationships were becoming less fraught, particularly with his parents and also with his former partner and child and her new husband. Some positive memories from his childhood, especially his relationship with his grandmother, seemed to suggest that there had been some early goodness that had later been lost in the layers of hate.

As his global hatred of humanity became fractured what emerged in its place was a more confusional state. He still hated the vast majority of the population but a more advanced ambivalence with significant others could be experienced and to some extent tolerated. From his depression emerged guilt at his previous brutal behaviour, especially towards the son of an ex-girlfriend and regarding the fact that he had later forced her to abort their child.

What can we say happened in this therapy? Can we say that from the hate emerged a form of love? Love seems like a fairly strong word to use but perhaps no other would do. Jonathan's attachment to others had been filled entirely with hate. Hate was awful, explosive and corrosive but gave him a passionate attachment to others. It was only with hate that he could have any relationships at all. Similarly, in the counter-transference, I found I could only reach him by my hate. He would not allow any other feeling to touch him, especially my fondness for him, only hate could form a link or attachment if I was expecting to reach him. But, and this is the point, it was only by really hating him that I could find any way to love him. Bollas (1985) describes a 'loving hate' that we can understand as an attempt to adapt relationships characterised by abuse or neglect. That is to say, hateful relating veiled behind a façade of giving love. I would like to suggest we can also think about hating-love: hating that is really about loving. In hating-love, we wish the best for the other precisely because we hate them and want, in effect, to help them be more lovable, perhaps for the selfish reason of wanting them to be lovable so we do not have to feel so bad about them. It seems to me that Jonathan and I established a deep and genuinely passionate relationship. First, this was by hate, then, once that connection had been made, we could explore other feelings. The therapy had a muta-tive effect (Carpy 1989; Strachey 1934) on both the analytic participants (Mann 1997). Mutual insight and understanding were gained when we could reflect on what we actually felt about each other.

This therapy ended when I left the institution I was working in. I think from the point of view of Jonathan's development, that was a premature end. I was confident that, had our work continued, his progress would have been greater. At the end he felt more contained, his relationships were less toxic, less hate based and more informed with insight and empathy towards others.

Discussion

It is the erotic that makes connections between people. As Freud puts it: 'Eros, which holds together everything in the world' (1921: 90). Eros forms links, creates bonds. Hate has more in common with Eros than Thanatos, it is part of the connecting principle rather than an aspect of disconnection and inertia. In that sense, hate can be thought of as libidinised aggression. We may say narcissism in general and pathological hate in misanthropy in particular can be conceived of as a self-preservative, although defensive, part of the life instinct. Although hate and destructiveness share much in common this should not automatically lead us to assume the operation of a death instinct, despite any manifest similarities. As I understand Thanatos, the death instinct, it is a drive towards disconnection, severance and complete and utter separation, in essence, a drive to achieve an inert, non-relational state, free from emotional attachments: the subject is effectively dead and therefore has no relationship to the object. Hatred may include a wish for death (to murder self or other) but, in itself, it is a form of connection. Hatred binds us to the object: it is Eros with poisoned arrows. That is to say, as a passion it brings us into a relationship with the other. Although hatred can be destructive and desires severance both the means and the end are relational.

Via the conduit of emotional attachment, it establishes a connection between the self and the hated object. We might describe hate as a perverse Eros. Stoller (1975) makes us aware that perversion is the erotic form of hatred; we might say, hatred is the destructive (or perverse) form of love. A statement like this needs instant clarification: all I mean to imply here is that love and hate are united by their capacity to form links. Desires, whether loving or hateful, bind us in relationships. Desires, whether cold or hot, are neither inert nor dead: they have a vitality. To have no desire is to break the connections that bind, to be severed from the relational: to be dead. It is distinct from the wish to kill or be killed, both of which are highly object related.

Hate, like love or the erotic, draws the patient and therapist into a passionate connection. With such a passionate connection we know they are inside us and we are inside them, thus the emotional distance of indifference is hardly in existence. I have written extensively about the erotic bond (Mann 1989, 1994, 1997, 1999, 2001). But hate, as distinct from love and the erotic has a peculiar fixity: as Blum (1997) notes, love can often turn into hate but rarely do we see hate turn into love. If I may paraphrase William Congreve's famous quote from *The Mourning Bride*: 'Heaven has no rage like love to hatred turned' we might also say Hell hardly needs to worry about hate to loving turned. This is the problem posed by hate disorders including the narcissistic personality when the personality is saturated by a dominion of hate it poses great therapeutic difficulties. How can therapy enable something good to exist in a psychological universe where hateful destructiveness prevails? Gabbard (1996) describes various technical approaches to malignant transference hate. Although he does not use the classification the patients he describes exhibit profound narcissistic personalities. His description that these patients bring a 'malignant trans-ference' to the therapy epitomises the therapeutic problem with these patients. Blum advocates a calm distance from hate. I consider this a com-mendable but a somewhat unrealistic idea: the nature of hate is that it forms a connection regardless of the distance. When the therapist tries to keep too great a distance from his or her own negative or hateful feelings, there is a danger that unconscious hate in the counter-transference is difficult to register.

It is primarily through loving relationships both as a child and adult that most people find opportunities for psychological growth. Yet love also implies helplessness. Freud (1930: 82) writes: 'We are never so defenceless against suffering as when we love; never so hopelessly unhappy as when we have lost our loved object or its love.' Hatred goes some way to main-taining the relationship to the loved object but seeks to control or punish it for the loss of love. Hate thereby keeps a connection, but at a safer distance so as to minimise helplessness. The narcissistic personality and the extreme form of misanthropy I have described, establish their relationships via the conduit of hate. In that respect, they are not yet ready to receive the therapist's love. The only connection that will initially establish a genuine relationship is with the therapist's hate. I think this might be the patient group that Winnicott (1947) refers to when he states that some patients actively seek our hate. Hate is a difficult feeling for therapists and goes against not only our attempts at neutrality but also our inner convictions that, both as professionals and as individuals, we are trying to do our best for the patient. Winnicott's concept of 'objective hate' has been seriously challenged (Blum 1997; Etchegoyen 1991) so I would doubt that many therapists, including Winnicott himself, can really hate anybody objectively. By its nature hate is a subjective experience. More feasible perhaps is the therapist's willingness to come to terms with the extent of their hate and to be prepared to hate the patient with a view to doing as little harm as possible and hopefully even some good. In so doing, it would be hoped that this kind of hating is new for the patient and gradually has a mutative effect on the misanthrope's internal world. I think of this as a hating-love. The therapist is not restraining his or her hate, which might be the only way the patient can establish a relationship, rather what is restrained is the therapist's desire to act destructively with the hate. Hartmann, Kris and Loewenstein (1949) and Anna Freud (1972) have also indicated that destructiveness in hate may only be tamed by self- and object love. Being less destructive, the therapist might then be in a better position to begin doing something more constructive and, more creative, perhaps finding some love, something lovable in the patient, maybe even about his or her own hatefulness.

A hating-love might not be so bad. With this in mind I think of two instances of hating-love. The first is the fictional account of Goethe's Faust where Mephistopheles does good:

'Say at last – who art thou?'
'That Power I serve
Which wills forever evil
Yet does forever good.'

The other example is the Truth and Reconciliation Tribunal in South Africa after apartheid where the hatred of racial division was processed by trying to understand rather than just blame. It would seem from this discussion that the patient needs to know the therapist can hate as well as love them. In some instances, the therapist's capacity to contain the hate in a loving way allows hatred to be modified and mollified; hatred can be transformed into something less than totally destructive.

Jonathan felt his life amounted to little because he had not had children. Although there was a daughter with a former partner, he suspected her fidelity and therefore doubted his paternal role. It seemed to me that whatever the truth about his ex-partner, Jonathan was not able to think of himself as a father because psychological factors prevented him from imagining himself as creative or procreative. Undoubtedly, this was also linked to his primal scene phantasies (Mann 1997: 138–61). To consider oneself creative has little to do with actually conceiving children but is more concerned with feeling that the self is capable of a 'supremely creative act' (Money-Kyrle 1968), which is very unlikely in a psyche filled with hate. The misanthrope's dilemma is that they cannot get out of the hating universe without the aid of another, a dependency that, in itself, is experienced as wounding and hateful. Yet with the therapist's hating-love there is an opportunity if not for love then at least a different, less toxic kind of hate.

Conclusion

I read Molière's comic masterpiece *The Misanthrope* to gain more insight into this condition. Alceste (the misanthrope) in the play, written in 1666, seemed to mirror my misanthropic patients. For example, the misanthrope's narcissistic grandiosity, hatred, lack of personal responsibility, the self-destructive willingness to suffer defeat in order to maintain a moral superiority, the wish for hermitage, the pollutive effect of any failing destroying all virtue, human insincerity, and so on. The comic factor was also shared: the extremity of views of Alceste and Jonathan often blurred the boundary between comedy and tragedy.

I am not familiar with Molière's complete *oeuvre* but the The *Misanthrope* seems different from a number of his other plays in that the last act is left in open-ended suspense. There is no theatrical resolution to the drama rounding off the story and tidying up the loose ends. Alceste wants to retreat into a rustic solitude away from the human race. His love, Celimene, refuses such a life of isolation. They argue, split up and leave the stage separately, the misanthrope determind to find his remote sanctuary. The last lines are spoken by their friends who wonder if they can do anything to persuade him to give up his foolish plan. The audience is left wondering whether Alceste and Celimene will ever reunite. I find this ambiguous uncertainty is like an echo or reflection of the therapeutic work with narcissistic personalities in which a positive therapeutic outcome is so uncertain. An effective outcome relies on the misanthrope's ability to experience something other than hate. This also requires therapists to be able to experience their own hate as well as their patients' hate, in a more creative, less destructive manner. This presents narcissistic patients with a potential for working through issues, although it remains uncertain as to whether they will be able to utilise these opportunities. Perhaps, in the tradition of Molière, it is appropriate to conclude these thoughts about misanthropy on such a note of uncertainty.

References

Blum, H.P. (1997) 'Clinical and developmental dimensions of hate', *Journal of the American Psychoanalytic Association* 45: 359–75

Bollas, C. (1985) 'Loving hate', *Annual of Psychoanalysis* 12/13: 221–373

Carpy, D.V. (1989) 'Tolerating the countertransference: a mutative process', *International Journal of Psychoanalysis* 70: 287–94

Chasseguet-Smirgel, J. (1984) *Creativity and Perversion*, London: Free Association Books

Etchegoyen, R.H. (1991) *The Fundamentals of Psychoanalytic Technique*, London: Karnac

Freud, A. (1972) 'Some comments on aggression', *International Journal of Psychoanalysis* 53: 163–71

Freud, S. (1918) 'The taboo of virginity. Contribution to the psychology of love', *Standard Edition 11*, London: Hogarth Press

—— (1921) 'Group psychology and the analysis of the ego', *Standard Edition 18*, London: Hogarth Press

—— (1930) 'Civilisation and its discontents', *Standard Edition 21*, London: Hogarth Press

Gabbard, G.O. (1993) 'On hate in love relationships: the narcissism of minor differences revisited', *Psychoanalytic Quarterly* 62: 229–38

—— (1996) *Love and Hate in the Analytic Setting*, Northvale, NJ: Jason Asonson

Goethe, J.W. (1986) *Faust*, Harmondsworth: Penguin

Graves, R. (1955) *The Greek Myths*, Harmonsworth: Penguin

Hartmann, H., Kris, E. and Loewenstein, R. (1949) 'Notes on the theory of aggression', *Psychoanalytic Study of the Child* 3/4: 9–36

Hess, J. (2000) quoted in 'I hate your guts – in a subtle way', *The Guardian*, 10 May, p. 4

Kernberg, O. (1974) 'Factors in the psychoanalytic treatment of narcissistic personalities', in *Essential Papers on Narcissism*, A. Morrison (ed.), New York and London: New York University Press

—— (1993) 'The psychopathology of hatred' in *Rage, Power and Aggression*, R. Glick and S. Roose (eds), New Haven, CT: Yale University Press

—— (1995) 'Hatred as a core affect of aggression' in *The Birth of Hatred*, S. Akhtar and S. Kramer (eds), Northvale, NJ: Jason Aronson

Kohut, H. (1966) 'Form and transformations of narcissism' in *Essential Papers on Narcissism*, A. Morrison (ed.), New York and London: New York University Press

Ledermann, R. (1987) 'Narcissistic disorder: a Jungian view of its aetiology and treatment', *British Journal of Psychotherapy* 3(4): 359–69

Mann, D. (1989) 'Incest: the father and the male therapist', *British Journal of Psychotherapy* 6: 143–53

—— (1994) 'The psychotherapist's erotic subjectivity', *British Journal of Psychotherapy* 10(3): 344–54

—— (1997) *Psychotherapy: An Erotic Relationship – Transference and Counter-transference Passion*, London: Routledge

—— (ed.) (1999) *Erotic Transference and Countertransference: Clinical Practice in Psychotherapy*, London: Routledge

—— (2001) 'Erotics and ethics: the passionate dilemmas of the therapeutic couple' in *Values and Ethics in the Practice of Psychotherapy and Counselling*, L. Murdin and F.P. Barnes (eds), Cambridge: Cambridge University Press

Molière (1959) *The Misanthrope and Other Plays*, Harmondsworth: Penguin

Money-Kyrle, R. (1968) 'Cognitive development' in *The Collected Papers of Roger Money-Kyrle*, Strath Tay: Clunie Press

Stoller, R. (1975) *Perversion: the Erotic Form of Hatred*, London: Marefield Library

Strachey, J. (1934) 'The nature of the therapeutic action of psychoanalysis', *International Journal of Psychoanalysis* 15: 127–59

Winnicott, D.W. (1947) 'Hate in the countertransference' in *Through Paediatrics to Psychoanalysis*, London: Hogarth Press

—— (1958) 'The capacity to be alone' in *The Maturational Processes and the Facilitating Environment*, London: Hogarth Press

—— (1971) 'The use of the object and relating through identification' in *Playing and Reality*, Harmondsworth: Penguin

Chapter 8

The victim's revenge: 'he is "crime" and I am "punishment"' (*Rigoletto*)[1]

Celia Harding

Introduction

Rigoletto sings these lines in Verdi's opera as he takes revenge on the Duke, for stealing and defiling his daughter, by arranging a contract on his life. The assassin asks Rigoletto for his name and the name of his victim. Rigoletto identifies his victim as crime and himself, the avenger, as punishment.

Revenge

This chapter is about revenge, the desire to inflict equivalent injury or damage in retaliation for wrongs or injury received (*Collins Concise Dictionary*). Psychoanalytically, revenge is both a primitive form of justice under 'talion law', 'an eye for an eye', and a primitive survival strategy, albeit one that is liable to backfire by provoking further retaliation. By perpetuating an increasingly vicious and intractable cycle, revenge is fundamentally dysfunctional and destructive. The embittered protagonists become victim and perpetrator in turn as each retaliatory attack provokes a response, escalating the damage and destruction and reducing the chances of resolution and reparation. This process is observable at all levels of human experience including international affairs:

> The Palestine question has degenerated into the grimmest kind of struggle, the sort in which both sides feel their national survival is at stake, and each shrinks from compromise lest the other construes it as a weakness or surrender. To an extent that is rare and frightening even for this long conflict, revenge and bloodlust are displacing rational political calculation.
>
> (*The Economist* 11 May 2002: 13)

---

1 This chapter originated from discussions on the theme of revenge by members of the Association for Psychotherapy in East London.

The victim

The perpetrator of revenge was once a victim. The victim desires revenge for trauma sustained at the hands of a perpetrator acting from 'weakness, ignorance or deliberate fault'. Traumatic experience overwhelms the victim's mental capacities to process them (Freud 1937: 22; 1940: 184f). Victims who have to manage their experiences as best they can without emotional support, may manage their helplessness by installing their experience as victim into the structure of their identity. They identify with 'the aggressor' and turn their passive, helpless position into an active repetition, courting injuries from their internal and external environment and then seeking revenge (Mollon 2002: 264). The mind's revenge organisation converts the terror of helplessness and loss into eroticised excitement, in a sado-masochistic solution to the pain of trauma and attendant core-complex anxieties. (Glasser 1996; Ruszczynski, Chapter 6, this volume).

The psychotherapist faces the question of how to work with the destructive rage of a patient whose internal world is organised around vengeance for actual, perceived or imagined injuries. The victimised patient needs the therapist to understand the impact of past traumatising experiences: therapists betray their patients when they fail to acknowledge the validity of past injuries. However, if it becomes apparent that a patient is turning inward on the self or outward onto others the injuries originally inflicted on them, the therapist who ignores this side of the equation equally betrays the patient. One obstacle to addressing the perpetrator in the victim is that the victim identity is founded on the victim's sense of their total innocence and of the perpetrator's total culpability. This makes it difficult for victims to recognise their complicity when they have recruited victimisation. Also to connect with the rage, pain and fear of helplessness behind their vengeful attacks on themselves and others.

The therapist needs to find ways to address both the traumatised enraged victim and the vengeful perpetrator in the patient's mind, the latter frequently appearing as a sadistic superego seeking revenge on a masochistic, victimised, ego. Jeremy Holmes neatly summarises the therapist's task:

> It is important to see the 'victim' of deprivation not as a passive recipient of stress, but as an active agent, in a dynamic relationship with his environment, trying to make sense of experience, to master it and to cope the best he can, but also, via the benign and vicious circles of neurosis, as an active participant in his own downfall or deliverance.
>
> (1993: 55)

Rigoletto

The story of 'Rigoletto' offers an archetypal representation of a victim's mind organised around revenge.

Rigoletto is a hunchback, the jester of the Duke of Mantua's Court. He encourages the Duke and his nobles in their depraved and licentious behaviour. As the opera begins, the court, under Rigoletto's orchestration, incites the Duke to seduce Ceprano's wife. Rigoletto mocks Ceprano's distress. The entrance of Monterone, whose daughter has already been seduced by the Duke, interrupts the scene. Rigoletto mocks and taunts Monterone until 'the old man' curses the Duke and Rigoletto. This curse haunts Rigoletto throughout the opera.

In stark contrast to the opulence of the court where he is jester, Rigoletto lives in poverty-stricken surroundings. In his impoverished, dark world he hides his daughter, Gilda, to protect her from contamination by the ostentatious and depraved world where he spends his days. Gilda's only outing is to church. The Duke sees her there and determines to seduce her.

The noblemen, led by Ceprano, discover Gilda's existence and mistake her for Rigoletto's mistress. They plan to abduct her to avenge Rigoletto for his part in abducting their wives for the Duke. Ceprano sweetens his revenge by drawing Rigoletto into the plot by convincing Rigoletto that their victim is another man's wife. Ceprano thereby hoists Rigoletto with his own petard. The plotters blindfold Rigoletto and he holds the ladder for them while they climb in the window to steal his daughter.

The distraught Rigoletto finds his daughter at the Duke's court. Gilda confesses her love for the Duke. Rigoletto blames his catastrophe on the old man's curse. Sparafucile, an assassin, presents himself as a possible agent to carry out Rigoletto's revenge on the Duke for corrupting his daughter. Sparafucile entices the Duke to his house with promises of his sister Maddalena's sexual favours. Rigoletto takes Gilda to witness the Duke's seduction of Maddalena in an attempt to disabuse her of her belief in the Duke's love. Although hurt by the Duke's infidelity, Gilda urges her father to forgive the Duke. She leaves the scene in great distress and Rigoletto finalises his revenge contract with Sparafucile.

Rigoletto seals his arrangement with Sparafucile to assassinate the Duke and leaves the scene planning to return later to dispose of the body. Meanwhile, Maddalena falls for the Duke's charms and objects to the plan to murder him. She and Sparafucile agree to spare the Duke and kill a stranger in his place, should one appear. Gilda returns disguised as a man and, overhearing the assassination plot and contingency plan, she knocks on the door and offers herself as the sacrificial stranger.

Rigoletto returns to relish his revenge by receiving and disposing of the Duke's body. As he contemplates the sack containing the body, he hears the Duke singing in the background. In the sack he finds his fatally wounded daughter. With her dying breath Gilda implores Rigoletto to forgive the Duke and herself. In anguish, Rigoletto cries: 'The curse is fulfilled.'

The revenge organisation

By the time we meet Rigoletto, it is difficult to distinguish between victim and perpetrator. In order to understand the convoluted, sado-masochistic revenge organisation, I will take it apart to examine its constituent parts with illustrations from Rigoletto.

The vulnerable self and victim armour

At the core of every victim and perpetrator is a vulnerable self, identified by Rosenfeld as the 'libidinal self'. The vulnerable self is characterised by being loving and lovable, caring and receptive and appreciative – it epitomises sanity because it is in touch with the reality of its needs for others (Rosenfeld 1987: 106). But if no empathic, protective object is available (Parsons & Dermen 1999) needing, loving and openness to others is dangerous to the vulnerable self and knowledge of the reality of the need for others is quashed (Kalsched 1996).

When victim experiences are managed by installing them as part of the person's identity, a distinction can be made between a familiar state of feeling victimised and the helpless, suffering vulnerable self. The victim identity functions as an emotional armour protecting the vulnerable self from exposure to the dangerous vicissitudes of life. The victim develops this armoury in reaction to early experiences of feeling traumatised and unprotected without empathic caretakers to recognise and respond to signals of distress. People cannot internalise a capacity to protect themselves, adequately and appropriately, when they have not experienced the reliable responsive presence of a protective object early in life (Parsons & Dermen 1999). When vulnerability with other people is dangerous, intimate relationships are avoided, and if one does expose oneself to danger and is hurt, punishing attacks on the self become part of a destructive 'self-care' system: 'the aggressive energies of the psyche are turned back upon the dependent aspects and we have an internal environment where self-attack for neediness is a constant occurrence' (Kalsched 1996: 23). Sometimes, I suggest, a victim identity forms part of that 'self-care system' that evolves to protect the person's vulnerable self from experiencing helplessness and the pain of betrayal, deprivation, neglect, and/or abuse.

Rigoletto

To connect with Rigoletto's vulnerability we need to imagine how his earliest relationship with his mother might have been. His mother gave birth to a baby with a physical deformity. Considering Rigoletto's story, it seems likely that she was traumatised by this experience, overwhelmed by the narcissistic injury of giving birth to a deformed infant, activating primitive anxieties that she had damaged him (Klein 1928, 1945). She may have been unable to think about her infant except through a highly distorted representation of him (Fonagy & Target 1995). The infant Rigoletto would then have perceived himself only as distorted and deformed. He may have sensed in her mind a terrifying hatred of him that threatened his infantile self, a hatred maybe experienced as mother's infanticidal wishes (Sinason 1997: 268). This horrifying view of himself would be too dreadful to contemplate, leaving him unable to think about other people's intentions and thoughts or his own. Thus his capacity to mentalise his feelings would become severely impaired, to be expressed instead through his body, his actions, his environment and, when he felt psychologically endangered, through violent aggression (Fonagy & Target 1995).

We can imagine that Rigoletto saw himself as doubly cursed: physically handicapped and unlovable, the victim of his mother's inability to think about him with love. This would leave him believing he was hated and hateful, badly wronged but also badly wrong, if not evil, inside. The sadistic malice and suffering masochism of his victim armoury expresses his conviction of hatefulness but may also feel justified as a revenge for his mother's hatred.

Paranoid-schizoid processes

Paranoid-schizoid processes form the structure that holds in place a mind organised around vengefulness. The self within the victim armour is actually vulnerable and helpless and as liable to become overwhelmed as it was at the time of the original traumatising experiences. People who need to resort to a victim armoury are unlikely to have received consistent empathic thoughtful responses to their distress, leaving them ill equipped to mentalise their distressing experiences for themselves (Fonagy 2001). Without the capacities necessary to develop a mind of one's own, experiences have to be organised in primitive ways such as splitting good from bad, right from wrong in extreme ways and relying on physical enactments and 'talion law' to restore narcissistic equilibrium. Such scaffolding provides a semblance of continuity and structure to the insubstantial, unmentalised sense of self.

The person armoured in a victim identity exists in an internal world of certainties, of black and white, where everything is either ideal or rotten. In idealisation, a person may be put beyond the reach of disappointment and abuse whereas denigrated people and situations lead to despair and destructive rage where all is spoiled but comfortingly familiar. In this state of mind, all is clear and simple: we know the score, who is who and what is what, nothing is unpredictable, nothing destabilises and exposes vulnerability. In particular, the victim identity is predicated on innocence of any destructive motives or impulses: these belong to perpetrators. Relationships are between perpetrators who pursue their own interests, using and abusing their victims ruthlessly. The victim of such misuse and abuse experiences trauma without the sting in its tail, a miserable but familiar situation. Without the delusion of this victim armour, the vulnerable self would be left terrifyingly helpless and utterly confused, in a fog without map or compass.

Rigoletto

The operatic setting of Rigoletto shows his internal world split between idealisation and denigration, good and bad, past and present, all kept rigorously apart; when this splitting begins to disintegrate, the structure of his mind collapses with it (Bergstein 2003). The opulence of the court where Rigoletto works contrasts sharply with the poverty-stricken surroundings where he lives. The handsome, able-bodied Duke contrasts starkly with Rigoletto's physical deformity. Rigoletto enviously attacks and perverts the idealised, able-bodied nobles, by inciting them to depravity. He hides Gilda, who represents his vulnerable, lovable and loving good self, to protect her from contamination by the world he has corrupted with his envy and vindictiveness. Rigoletto protects Gilda from his hate-filled history, refusing to tell her his name. He restricts her access to the outside world, only allowing her to leave the house to attend church. Gilda can be seen as representing Rigoletto's vulnerability and innocence he wishes he had. As such, she is hidden away in an attempt to protect the unblemished part of himself from terrifying realities. But when the splits begin to break down, as they do after the Duke seduces Gilda, we see how Rigoletto's strategy backfires: in protecting Gilda from reality he has deprived her of opportunities to learn from experience about the realities of life and relationships. And so she remains naively vulnerable, and susceptible to the Duke's advances.

Secondary victimisation

The deprived child feels angry with the person who failed them. When the neglectful, failing or abusive caretaker is unable to respond empathically to the child's angry protest, the child comes to expect retaliation and rejection in reaction to their rage. This may initiate a tendency to store a backlog of rage while seeking opportunities to express it covertly.

'Secondary victimisation' is one outlet for the victim's hidden rage. I adopt this idea from the concept of 'secondary handicap' developed by Sinason in her work with handicapped patients who defensively exaggerated their impairment when they were unable to face unbearable realities associated with it (Sinason 1992: 18–23). They compounded their primary disability by hijacking their impairment to express their disturbing feelings and impulses.

When a victim's unexpressed rage becomes organised in a revenge structure, the damage of the original injury may be compounded by secondary victimisation. This creates a disguised way to express the rage that victims feel about their injuries, avenging themselves by maintaining and exacerbating their wounds. Secondary victimisation also inflicts revenge on whoever is thought to be the perpetrator by implying that the damage caused is irremediable. Freud describes this internal situation and its repercussions in melancholia:

> The patients usually still succeed, by the circuitous path of self-punishment, in taking revenge on their original object and in tormenting their loved one through their illness, having resorted to it in order to avoid the need to express their hostility to him openly.
>
> (Freud 1917: 251)

In secondary victimisation, the sufferers' rage and destructiveness towards themselves for being vulnerable and towards those who failed to protect them, concentrates around their injury. They identify with the aggressor, further injuring themselves by perpetuating and magnifying their wounded state. At the same time, they identify with the helpless suffering victim. The wound they once passively received they now actively keep open, by continuing to do to themselves what they perceive to have been done to them. If they were aware of this double identification, they would be exposed to raw vulnerability and grief for the losses caused by the primary and secondary victimisation.

Victims of past tragedies and crimes are sometimes reported in the media as saying 'they have ruined my life forever'. When this has become an entrenched conviction, unconsciously maintained in a highly destructive and vengeful way, it typifies a secondary victim's armoury. Experiences of ill-treatment provide some victims with outlets for their unconscious rage at their original injury in the only form consistent with the victim identity: justification for their sense of grievance and righteous rage. Contrariwise, experiences of kindness and understanding may be rejected if these feel inconsistent with the victim identity or liable to dilute it.

Rigoletto

Rigoletto has chosen to be a professional jester thereby inviting others to victimise him for their entertainment. The role of court jester provides Rigoletto with the perfect victim armoury to protect his vulnerable self while providing an outlet to express the destructive rage he feels about his situation. As court jester he caricatures the distorted image of himself that he saw in his mother's eyes (Fonagy & Target 1995), thereby attacking both himself and his mother with a self-image that, he believes, sentenced him to be hated and hateful all his life.

Repetition compulsion

Freud maintained that we repeat in actions the experiences that we cannot bear to remember (Freud 1914: 150), identifying the repetition compulsion as an aspect of the destructive instinct (1920: 21f). More recent understanding of the developmental origins of the repetition compulsion suggest that children who are consistently treated neglectfully by their caretaker as though they had no thoughts or feelings of their own, are unlikely to develop the capacity to reflect on their experiences. While this protects them from conscious exposure to their emotions and fantasies that might overwhelm them, it exposes them to the risk of repeating the traumatising experience:

> Although restriction of mentalisation was originally adaptive, there is a clear and powerful link between this restricted capacity and vulnerability to later trauma. The inability to reflect upon the mental state of the perpetrator, as well as the reaction of the self, may prevent the child from resolving the original traumatic experience or coping with subsequent assault.
>
> (Fonagy 2001: 176)

People who are unable to bear the knowledge of their vulnerability are bound to go on repeating their original trauma. They find themselves drawn, with the 'random precision'[2] of unconscious processes, to situations and relationships in which they re-enact their painful experiences in one form or another and feel victimised again.

When in the grip of the repetition compulsion, victims are complicit in their own suffering. The compulsion to repeat a painful experience can serve several purposes. It can be a way of giving expression to, and thus disposing of, overwhelming feelings, particularly destructive impulses, which cannot be mentally processed and symbolised (Fonagy 2001). It can serve as a corrective punishment, on behalf of the destructive 'self-care' system, for exposing the self to suffering and a reminder that vulnerability is dangerous. This may reinforce the victim identity as a protection for the endangered self from the threat of helplessness and overwhelming distress. The repetition may be an attempt to master a traumatising situation and the feelings evoked, particularly helplessness.

---

2 This expression comes from Pink Floyd's 'Shine on You Crazy Diamond', *Wish You Were Here*, 1975.

Victims may express their vengeful impulses by 'mindlessly' exposing themselves to risk of further victimisation. However, even when victims have unconsciously orchestrated their own downfall, the real consequences will differ from the phantasy of secondary gains that the disaster may have been designed to achieve (Garland 1998). People risk becoming re-traumatised when they are driven to invite a repetition of harm: no matter how familiar, the re-experience of the trauma can overwhelm again. From the point of view of therapy, when the patient's victim armour has been penetrated by re-traumatisation, the therapist needs first to acknowledge the patient's actual vulnerability and suffering. Thereafter, the therapist may be able to help the patient to recognise the unconscious destructive impulses expressed through their complicity with this latest injury.

Rigoletto

In Rigoletto's story, we see the tragedy of the repetition compulsion writ large. As court jester, Rigoletto incites the hatred he saw in his mother's eyes and enacts his identification with that hatefulness. Unconsciously, he sabotages his wish to protect his good object when he assists in Gilda's abduction. These events merely confirm his victim identity as one who is cursed because Rigoletto lacks the mentalising capacities needed to use these experiences to make some progress towards the complexity and development of the depressive position. Instead, he avenges himself by arranging the Duke's murder and propels himself into a worse trauma. His revenge catastrophically backfires and Gilda is murdered in the Duke's place. Rigoletto destroys his good object, albeit by proxy, but this is too overwhelming for him to face. In the original play, on which the opera was based, the jester realises in anguish that he has killed his own daughter (Newman 1928: 43). But Rigoletto cannot bear this realisation even momentarily. The survival of his fragile mind would be jeopardised by his grief for his loss, and guilt for his part in causing it. Therefore, Rigoletto maintains himself as the victim of a curse, a condensation of his mother's perceived curse on him as an infant and his perpetuation of it through his identification with it (Fonagy & Target 1995).

Forgiveness and reparation: loosening the revenge organisation

Before Gilda dies, and indeed, earlier in the opera, she begs Rigoletto to forgive. As the representation of goodness, Gilda intuitively understands that forgiveness and reparation are the way forward, but her ignorance of reality prevents her from understanding that her father is not psychologically equipped to take this step. Rigoletto protected Gilda from knowing about the violence that was done to him during his lifetime and the violence he subsequently did to himself and others in order to survive. The capacity to forgive and repair is achievable only after working through the conflicts and anxieties that underlie each component of the revenge structure and facing the attendant guilt and loss.

To the mind dominated by paranoid-schizoid processes, something bad must remain irreparable and unforgivable because it cannot be undone and made as good as new (Rey 1996). To forgive and allow some repair of the damage done seems to exonerate the perpetrator by implying that what they did was not so bad after all: if an injury is forgivable it suggests that no real harm was done.

In order to overcome this impasse, patients dominated by paranoid-schizoid processes have to become able to risk experiencing their vulnerability in their therapy, in order to discover in their therapist an empathic protective person who can think about them and embody a tolerant, understanding superego. This discovery is a cumulative process that may take years to develop. It enables patients to gradually internalise, for themselves, a protective, thoughtful and forgiving superego that can counter and modify attacks from their destructive 'self-care system' and allow their victim armoury to be dismantled safely. They are then more able to face their guilt and grief for the damage they have done to themselves and others. These developments can only occur alongside shifts in the paranoid-schizoid structure of the mind:

> Forgiveness requires us to recognise the co-existence of good and bad feelings, sufficient badness to justify guilt, and sufficient goodness to deserve forgiveness. We need to believe this is true of ourselves and also of our objects. The wish to exact revenge must be recognised, and responsibility for the damage we have done to our objects has to be accepted. This means that to be forgiven, bad elements in our nature have to be accepted but sufficient good feeling must exist for us to feel regret and the wish to make reparation.
>
> (Steiner 1993: 85)

Patients have to recognise how their victim identity has functioned as a protective armoury and risk, often for the first time, exposing the protected, but imprisoned vulnerable self to the vagaries of reality in their therapy. Reparation entails forgiving the perpetrator, accepting the perpetrator's humanity, which includes their capacity to be destructive whether through 'ignorance, weakness or deliberate fault' (Steiner 1993). This becomes possible when victims accept the reality of their own human weakness and fallibility and their own responsibility for protecting and understanding themselves and their needs.

The compulsion to repeat can begin to lose its grip when the pain, guilt and loss from being hurt can be thought about and realistic reparation becomes an acceptable recompense. Without the capacity to accept a partial repair, the need to repeat is compulsive and the vicious cycle continues (Rey 1996: 208).

The example of Ms B

Ms B has experienced during her lifetime more than an expectable quota of accidents, violating experiences and tragedies in the context of an unresponsive and unempathic environment. She had reason to see herself as a victim and, like others with similar histories, made sense of her lot by believing that she was essentially rotten and deserved bad treatment. At the same time she was convinced that she was special, deserving privilege and success. She oscillated between these two extreme self-perceptions.

André Green captures the essential core of Ms B's revenge organisation when he writes:

> If we wish to pay attention to what it is that enrages us about being dropped on this earth, all fucked up . . . we might place the accent on the other, upon whom we depend. This consoles us, for in this instance – at least – there is a solution to hand. Otherwise, we might focus on the power of vengefulness, because far from correcting the 'irregularity' which affects us, the inadequacy of the other's response aggravates it further.
>
> (2001: 69)

Ms B did not ask to be born and wished for an exit door from life: 'Life is hard and then you die.' This disguised the fact that she baulked at engaging with the reality of life's struggles and had not renounced her search for an ideal mother to make everything right. She came to therapy expecting a fairy godmother with a magic wand and realised she was still waiting long after she had intellectually recognised that I was not going to oblige. She hated reality, particularly the reality that she was vulnerable and could not expect other people to protect her interests. She saw herself as the victim of other people's self-interest both when she was and when she was not. This conviction surfaced particularly vividly in our relationship when I raised with her the possibility of writing and publishing a professional paper based on some of the work we had done together.

Ultimately, Ms B blamed her mother for life's harsh realities. After nearly 10 years in therapy Ms B remained driven to take revenge on her mother, whom she blamed for her unhappiness. Her deepening understanding of her mother's hostility and emotional neglect towards her as a young child seemed to have yielded no compassion or forgiveness towards her mother or herself.

We came to understand that her carelessness towards herself was partly her identification with the emotionally neglectful and unprotective mother and partly her way of showing her mother what she had done to her. To Ms B taking care of herself was tantamount to letting her mother 'off the hook' for neglecting her childhood needs. Unconsciously, her achievements equally signified exonerating her mother, denying the permanent and devastating effect of the actual and imagined injuries her mother's negligence had caused or exacerbated. Ms B was an enterprising and imaginative woman whose achievements fell well below her capabilities. In both the mundane and special aspects of her life, when she did allow herself to attain her goals, she resisted actions required to maintain and build on her achievements. In both her private and her work life, she often felt cheated of the benefits of her efforts. Both her achievements and her failures seemed to reignite her hatred towards her mother (and towards me, in the transference) triggering a vengeful backlash. As we came to understand the vengeful nature of her attacks on herself, her mother and her therapist, the scaffolding holding her revenge organisation in place gradually loosened.

The victim armoury defending and imprisoning the vulnerable self

Ms B returned from a break, more determined than ever to finish therapy. She bombarded me with arguments as to why her therapy should end. This shifted when we were able to connect with her terror of acknowledging her need of me. Having been able to allow herself an awareness of her neediness and vulnerability, she recognised with remorse her propensity to spot an 'open wound' in others and 'poke sticks in it'. She was recognising how unconsciously she had turned her unbearable fear of helplessness into sadistic, sexualised power. She saw how she attacked others to pre-empt any attempts they might make to exploit chinks in her armour. This realisation, and the working through that followed, enabled her to register when she was feeling threatened by intimacy and to contain her impulse to lash out and distance the other. Intense 'core complex anxieties' lay at the heart of her vulnerability, hidden beneath her revengeful sado-masochistic way of relating to herself and others (Glasser 1996).

Paranoid-schizoid processes of black and white certainties

Ms B was dominated by an inner world of idealisation and denigration, both of herself and others, oscillating between these two states of mind. This created a scaffold for her amorphous sense of self. We came to understand that her sense of agency and her capacity to think for herself had been chronically restricted by a highly regimented upbringing. In the absence of a mind of her own, she structured her mind with a system of rules and certainties. In her view, the participants in relationships had conflicting interests and gain for one automatically meant the other's loss. There was no middle ground where interests could be shared, a compromise reached and a mutually beneficial outcome achieved. She often saw herself as some-one else's tool with no say of her own. In her relationship with me, as with others, one of us was the weak supplicant exploited by the powerful other. When she began to realise that things were not so simple or certain, she had to face and endure terrifying uncertainty. She was actually vulnerable without her 'rules' and certainties until she developed a mind of her own with which to reflect on and process her experiences.

The primitive structure provided by paranoid-schizoid processes also restricted her mind severely. She punished her failing objects, and protected herself from confusion and further betrayal, by rejecting the possibility that people could change their minds. When her mother tried to show Ms B more affection as an adult, she rejected her: 'It's too late.' She was equally hard on herself. She found it hard to make decisions partly because once made, they were set in concrete. When things went wrong, she assumed she deserved to suffer for getting it wrong: 'You made your bed, you lie on it.' To change her mind felt like failure and weakness. In discussions about her wish to reduce her sessions or end her therapy, for example, she found it difficult to change her mind after we had reached some understanding of the feelings behind her wishes. To amend her original plan meant over-coming her sense of failure, of being weak and prey to my power. Even-tually, she was able to work towards leaving therapy over an extended period of time with a more open mind.

Managing destructiveness and rage by secondary victimisation

Whenever things went wrong, Ms B. tended to retreat into her victim armoury. She would drown out the pain of her vulnerable self with a deluge of familiar self-pity along the lines of: 'It always happens: whenever I have something someone takes it, controls it or spoils it.' We came to realise that whenever she felt failed or betrayed she vented her rage by unconsciously instigating an internal vandal or sniper to cause her accidents, sometimes incurring severe physical damage and emotional pain. On a more everyday level, when something went wrong – like oversleeping or a punctured tyre – she would 'know' that the whole day, and probably the whole week, would be ruined. And so it was! Gradually, she became more able to differentiate between the times when she was suffering from unavoidable misadventures, from the times when she was misused by others and from the times when she suffered because she had targeted herself with some vengeful destruc-tiveness. She came to recognise that she did need to be extra vigilant about taking care of herself, not only by taking realistic protective measures but also by taking into account the angry revengeful part of her that was secretly seeking opportunities to sabotage her. This enabled her to engage more with reality and find ways to rectify things rather than bingeing on junk food while slumped mindlessly in front of the television.

Repetition compulsion

Ms B frequently felt used and abused by her friends and in her work. She felt she had been robbed of many opportunities during her life. Her business achievements repeatedly failed to reflect her talents and new business ventures collapsed. We began to identify some of the booby traps she laid to satisfy her unconscious need to fail and keep her victim identity intact and her mother 'on the hook'. We realised that she tended to enter business relationships with 'crooks' likely to cheat her. She frequently felt that others benefited from her work and ideas, at her expense, in her business and her personal relationships and eventually in her therapy when I raised the possibility of my writing about our work. She seemed unable to renounce her illusion that others would look after her. To her surprise she found herself angrily saying one day: 'Why should I look after myself?' She needed to face the pain of betrayal when figures in the past had failed to protect her. She also needed to recognise her own complicity in betrayals in the present and her failure to protect herself. That she was able, finally, to permit me to write about our work together testified to her discovery that she could gain deeper understanding of herself from working with this evidence of my self-interest, enabling her to share without feeling robbed.

Reparation and forgiveness

As Ms B worked through the components of her revenge mentality, she began to find herself more able to face and engage with reality rather than taking cover in her victim armoury. She was awed by her discovery of contentment in ordinariness, no longer oscillating between spectacular wretchedness and brilliance. Allowing herself to have good things and to feel more secure and happy, activated anxieties about 'paying the price' and losing what she had found. She began to see how she had been 'hooked on suffering', detecting in that familiar state the intensity and 'rush' of sexual feelings: in effect, that she had sexualised her helplessness, pain and fear of loss by turning it into a dread-full excitement.

She began to allow herself more intimacy with her friends and became more able to restrain her impulse to 'throw stones' and 'poke sticks' to keep people at a distance when they felt too close. Ms B had been suspicious of and punitive towards children whom she perceived as devious and mercenary. Now she saw them as vulnerable, needing love, empathy and protection and she treasured her relationships with them. She discovered tolerance towards her mother's failings and became able to treat her with kindness, compassion and thoughtfulness. She movingly told me that through therapy she had found that she could love and be lovable. Reparation of the damage done to her by herself and others had begun.

Ms B's example shows how reparation has a particular meaning in the context of renouncing revenge as a solution. She reached a point when she could register that she had been hurt and could choose how to respond: to switch into a revenge reaction or to make a reparative move. Reparation began when she chose not to express her rageful pain by reflex revenge reactions. Instead, she became able to think about and process what had happened, protecting herself and the other from her vengeful reactions, identifying her own part in the situation and relating to the other's vulnerability. By restraining her destructive impulses for revenge, Ms B repaired some of her internal damage. By taking responsibility for intervening in the vicious revenge cycle, she made reparation to herself and her internal objects. Her love and compassion was liberated to heal her wounds, restoring her faith in the strength of her own love and lovability.

Ms B compared her inner world to the streets of Belfast before and after 'the Troubles'. It was as if she had been existing in a barricaded street and afraid that whenever she broke cover the sniper-within would shoot her down. Now she lived freely in an open street without barricades. She was vulnerable, but less at risk now that the internal sniper was in abeyance and open to negotiation, and now that she knew about asking people for help when needed. Paradoxically, her greater awareness of her vulnerability put her in a better position to look after herself.

It would be misleading to suggest that Ms B freed herself entirely from the power that her revenge mentality exerted over her mind. Part of her achievement in therapy was that she came to terms with the limits of her influence over the destructive sides of her, variously identified as the sniper, the vandal, the ogre or saboteur in her, liable to attack and damage the good things she had won (Kalsched 1996: 26). She came to accept that although she could not eradicate her destructive impulses, she could recognise them and check their power over her by not exaggerating and exacerbating their effects.

Secondary victimisation in everyday life or 'cutting off one's nose to spite one's face'

In conclusion, I briefly consider a relatively mild, but nevertheless destructive, form of the revenge organisation commonly activated in reaction to the injustices of everyday life. This is less a pervasive dominating mental organisation and more a transitory state of mind, a strategy to deal with rage about injustices, disappointments or injuries. Although this aggrieved state of mind is comparatively mild, it is nevertheless driven by destructive motives with destructive consequences. It is activated when people believe they have been wronged and unfairly treated. Instead of sorting out, and coming to terms with, their grievance, they harbour it in resentful rage. Identifying with the aggressor, turning passive into active, they direct their angry destructiveness at themselves by perpetuating the unfairness on themselves thereby keeping themselves in the victim's position – deprived, wronged, unjustly treated. They express their rage at feeling wronged by compounding the damage they perceive to have been inflicted on them. Simultaneously they punish the perceived perpetrator through the persistence and magnification of their suffering: 'Look what you've done to me.' This is colloquially known as 'cutting off one's nose to spite one's face':

> It transpired that Mr G refused to wear a helmet when riding his bike. He reasoned that cyclists who wear helmets encourage drivers to be careless. He was shocked to realise the price he was unconsciously prepared to pay – possibly his life – to teach the negligent driver a lesson. It became clear that, among other things, the careless driver stood for the negligence he ascribed to his parents for leaving him to fend for himself as a 'latchkey kid'.

References

Bergstein, M. (2003) 'Verdi's Rigoletto: The dialectic interplay of psychic positions in seemingly mindless violence', *International Journal of Psychoanalysis* 84(5): 1295–314

Fonagy, P. (2001) *Attachment Theory and Psychoanalysis*, New York: The Other Press

Fonagy, P. and Target, M. (1995) 'Understanding the violent patient: the use of the body and the role of the father' in *Psychoanalytic Understanding of Violence and Suicide*, R. Perelberg (ed.), London and New York: Routledge

Freud, S. (1914) 'Remembering, repeating and working through', *Standard Edition 12*, London: Hogarth Press

—— (1917) 'Mourning and melancholia', *Standard Edition 14*, London: Hogarth Press

—— (1920) 'Beyond the pleasure principle', *Standard Edition 18*, London: Hogarth Press

—— (1937) 'Analysis, terminable and interminable', *Standard Edition 23*, London: Hogarth Press

—— (1940) 'The outline' *Standard Edition 23*, London: Hogarth Press

Garland, C. (1998) *Understanding Trauma: A Psychoanalytical Approach*, London and New York: Karnac

Glasser, M. (1996) 'Aggression and sadism in the perversions' in *Sexual Deviation*, 3rd edn, I. Rosen (ed.), Oxford: Oxford University Press

Green, A. (2001) *The Chains of Eros*, London: Karnac

Holmes, J. (1993) *John Bowlby and Attachment Theory*, Hove and New York: Brunner-Routledge

Kalsched, D. (1996) *The Inner World of Trauma. Archetypal Defences of the Personal Spirit*, New York and London: Routledge

Klein, M. (1928) 'Early stages of the Oedipus Complex' in *Love, Guilt and Reparation and Other Works*, London: Routledge

—— (1945) 'The Oedipus Complex in the light of early anxieties' in *Love, Guilt and Reparation and Other Works*, London: Routledge

Mollon, P. (2002) *Remembering Trauma*, 2nd edn, Chichester and New York: John Wiley & Sons

Newman, E. (1928) *Stories of the Great Operas and their Composers*, New York: Dorset Press

Parsons, M. and Derman, S. (1999) 'The violent child and adolescent' in *Handbook of Child and Adolescent Psychotherapy*, M. Lanyado and A. Horne (eds), London and New York: Routledge

Rey, H. (1996) 'Reparation in universals of psychoanalysis' in *The Treatment of Psychotic and Borderline States*, London: Free Association Books

Rosenfeld, H. (1987) 'Destructive narcissism and the death instinct' in *Impasse and Interpretation*, London and New York: Routledge

Sinason, V. (1992) *Mental Handicap and the Human Condition*, London: Free Association Books

—— (1997) 'Gender-linked issues in psychotherapy with abused and learning disabled female patients' in *Female Experience*, J. Raphael-Leff and R. Jozef Perelberg (eds), London and New York: Routledge

Steiner, J. (1993) 'Revenge, resentment, remorse and reparation' in *Psychic Retreats*, London and New York: Routledge

Chapter 9

Bullying, education and the role of psychotherapy

John Woods

Introduction: the bully in context

From nasty little incidents in the nursery playground to the chronic problems of international relations, it seems that the abuse of power and the exploitation of others in the form of bullying is a ubiquitous characteristic of human nature. The word 'bully' in the *Oxford English Dictionary* has an interesting ancestry, which lies in an Old High German word, also found in modern Dutch, *boele* meaning lover or sweetheart. It is to be found in Shakespeare, where, for example, the much loved King is referred to as 'my bully boy' (Henry V Act 4, sc 1: 44) and it still exists in some old seafaring songs. At first this seems to make no sense until we think about the relationships between bullies and victims as forms of attachment based on the coercion and power of one person over another. The person who is ready to be a victim appears to be looking for someone who may make them suffer, just as the bully appears to be seeking out a victim. In this chapter, I argue that both bullies and victims seek to establish and maintain the sort of relationships that they have experienced from their earliest attachments.

Psychotherapists are often asked for help by other professions, teachers, social workers, who are facing behavioural problems of young people, aggression, violence, disruptive and delinquent behaviour, much of which can be summed up in the term bullying. But this raises a number of questions and problems of combining different perspectives. Often encounters between professionals who have very different tasks are unproductive. Education and psychotherapy are in some ways contradictory, the one being more focused on the transmission of knowledge about the world, the other focusing on spontaneous expressions of internal reality. If the role of the therapist is primarily to treat individuals, what relevance can this have for the management of the school environment, adolescent unit or children's home? Violence, designed as it usually is to assert power and prevent questioning, would seem to be the antithesis of education. But can education provide an antidote to the destructiveness in human nature? Part of the task of education is socialisation, but sometimes the social climate of the school becomes a microcosm of wider social conflicts. It has been widely recognised that authoritarian structures can be harmful to young children (Waddell 2002). But one consequence of doubts about the value of authoritarian structure is to increase uncertainty about the use of authority; this may be as damaging as the authoritarianism that is avoided.

In this chapter, I will explore the potential usefulness of the psychoanalytic perspective for promoting understanding and treatment of bullying in the wider social context, in particular, the school and the value to psychotherapists of what can be learned from the social contexts of individuals.

The social perspective

Adults are usually expected to have more power than children, which, in healthy situations, they use for mutual benefit or common good rather than to dominate others. However, from the Milgram experiments in the 1960s (reported in Fromm 1973: 80–86) to the recent torture of prisoners by the Allied soldiers 'bringing democracy' to Iraq (and all that has gone on between) there can be no doubt about the perpetual vulnerability of people to abuse their power.

In order to work with the problem it is necessary to look at the quality of the interaction between bully and victim. What is bullying? This is not a theoretical question since in specific situations, an alleged perpetrator will often claim that he was defending himself, not bullying. Equally problematic is that victims will often not admit to being bullied. Children may keep the shameful experience of being terrorised secret for a long time sometimes with disastrous consequences. The use of violence may be covert. Threats may be so subtle and coded that they are overlooked by an observer while clearly understood by the victim. Bullying can be understood as the consistent and compulsive exercise of power by one party over another. Coercion is common to all experiences of bullying. People who are bullied are deprived of their right to say no. Victims are under the power of others, silenced by the unequal relationships in which they are locked. A most chilling and convincing portrayal of such a locked relationship is to be found in Susan Hill's novel *I'm the King of the Castle*, in which one boy completely dominates another, thereby protecting himself from feelings of jealousy, envy and loss.

Research by the Youth Justice Department reported in *The Observer* (12 October 2003) found that 60 percent of all school children are anxious about being bullied in or around school; 20 percent of Glasgow schoolchildren carry weapons. Sixteen children committed suicide in 2002 in circumstances believed to be connected with their having been bullied. Sir Charles Pollard, Head of Youth Justice Board and a former Chief Constable, reportedly suggested that a permanent police presence is necessary in some schools. Seemingly isolated examples of extreme violence, such as the cases in the stabbings that are regularly reported in the media, usually occur in the context of a general bullying culture (*The Observer*, 12 October 2003).

As a therapist working in educational settings, I have occasionally been asked my opinion about whether bullying between young people is 'worse than it used to be'. In my view, young people do seem to be exposed to increasing levels of violence in their lives. Accompanying reports of pervasive bullying in schools, there is a tremendous amount of violence pumped into virtually every home by mass culture, i.e. by the adult world of big business. By the same token, our disregard for the destruction of the physical world is matched by a wilful blindness to the corrosive mental effects of many current aspects of popular culture. Film blockbusters, such as *The Matrix* or *The Lord of the Rings*, convey an underlying message that violence is the way to achieve one's goals. It is no wonder that youngsters assume that they can get what they want by violent means. And this is intricately bound up with sex. Sex sells, anything, to younger and younger children, whose need for acceptance and status in the peer group is exploited. Rape is commonplace in TV and film. Pornography is widely available as never before. 'Action movies' and video games show ever more exciting and effective ways of killing and maiming. Violence and sex become inextricably linked in the electronic world of visual/mental stimulation and this translates to the social world. Forcing someone to have sex, for example, has been reported as rife in some deprived subcultures such as housing estates around Paris. Undoubtedly, there are those who are more susceptible than others to the allure of instant gratification through the media. Typically, it will be those sections of society with less hope of the goodies promised by advertising and in those families who struggle to contain levels of frustration and domestic violence. The recent stream of 'reality' television shows, for example *Big Brother*, provides children with powerful invitations to join in the excitement of the violence depicted; and yet the vast majority are excluded from the glamour and adulation accorded to newly created 'celebrities'. Teachers are also concerned about the insidious effects of jealousy, rivalry and backbiting that is the staple content of some television 'soaps', which often erupt into hostile interactions between children.

In February 2002 in a Midlands town called Goole, a 35-year-old man called Danny Tandy kidnapped and tortured, over a period of 48 hours, a teenager who was suspected of stealing drugs and money. A number of his associates came and went, some of whom joined in the cutting, burning and beating. Accounts of the crime reveal some significant characteristics: playing pop music to the victim while mutilating his ears and other body parts was a deliberate imitation of the film *Reservoir Dogs*. This is reminiscent of the imitations of the *Clockwork Orange* assaults and murders that caused Stanley Kubrick to withdraw the film from general release. The more deep-rooted precipitating factor behind this atrocity was the family background of the main perpetrator, which was characterised by high levels of domestic violence by the father. Gilligan (1996) has documented masses of evidence to show that virtually all violent criminals have been brutalised by cruelty in their family background. And it comes as no surprise that all the people serving life sentences who contributed to a BBC television programme, *Lifers* by Rex Bloomstein (2004), had been abused or abandoned or both in the early years. The repetition of abuse seems inescapable in such cases.

Were things better 45 years ago? When, at the age of 11 I arrived in my North London Catholic grammar school, I was surprised to find that bullying and mugging were daily events. Looking back I can see that my strategy, quite spontaneously, was to ensure that I belonged to a small group of peers on whom I could depend for safety, because bullies, like predators, only go for those obviously weaker than themselves. A semblance of order was kept throughout the school by religious staff and teachers partly through measured use of physical punishment with the slipper and the cane and by the notable presence of a much feared deputy head renowned for his rages, when he had been known to throw boys against the wall. I believe that the terror of violence spinning out of control was a factor behind the general brutalising attitudes towards pupils. My survival strategy, built on the good fortune of having come from a non-abusive family, and on the trust that somehow or other I would find safety, was perhaps my first experience of the importance of the group, as essentially my new family. My personal experience, of course, did nothing to change the underlying ethos of the school.

Perhaps in those days many children suffered in silence. Today there are efforts to listen to young people. Each school is obliged to have an anti-bullying policy. Even so, an underlying law of the jungle persists in the playground, corridors and outside the school gates, beyond the reach of adult authority. With more open communication the failures of adult authority become increasingly obvious. William Golding's *Lord of the Flies*, written about the time of my own schooldays, effectively shows, I think, the liberation of violence in young people exposed to a combination of the absence of protective figures together with the pernicious use of power by adults. It is no accident that the sadistic gang in the story are formed from an elite group of public school boys. The potentially democratic and more egalitarian group came from more ordinary backgrounds: as day boys from grammar schools they were regarded as inferior, perhaps unconsciously envied by the public school boarders for their family life. All sides were ensnared in their predisposing mindsets, portrayed by the story's location on an island from which there was no escape. By contrast, in Susan Hill's *I'm the King of the Castle*, the part played by the failure of adult authority is more in the foreground, with parents so preoccupied by their own problems that they are blind to the destructive processes going on between their children.

The question arises as to whether the psychotherapist can effectively intervene in a social context. Even though psychological processes operate within the individuals involved, can a psychological approach make any difference to such a pronounced feature of the social environment? Is the psychotherapist as powerless as someone trying to reconcile national leaders at war or as irrelevant as applying first aid to the innumerable gross injuries of a battlefield? The psychotherapist's contribution comes from understanding the context: apparently meaningless events suddenly seem to make more sense when the underlying factors are understood. For example, the massacre at Columbine High School took place in a perfectly respect-able community. However, the main local employer was the largest weapons manufacturer in the world. This is shown in Michael Moore's film *Bowling for Columbine*, which examines the underpinning of violence in western culture. Brutal domination permeates society whether it takes place on a housing estate, in an educational establishment, or the workplace or on the international stage. Whereas some organisations aspire to a culture of fairness, freedom of speech, and creativity, others are ridden with feelings of persecution, fear, an ethos of 'protect your back, don't trust anyone, get them before they get you'. In my view, bringing together social and psy-chological perspectives can make a positive contribution to interventions into such social settings.

The psychotherapist's perspective

The psychotherapist's template is early relationships. The parent–infant relationship is an unequal one. Good parenting means negotiating this inequality by being open to the infant's communications. Parents sometimes feel bullied by their infants and if this persists it could lead to the parent bullying their dependent child. In a 'good-enough' situation as Winnicott (1962: 67) called it, there is a constant process of negotiation between the needs of parent and infant. Even if mother–infant interpretations seem remote from the bullying that occurs in the world, a universal principle of equal rights and communication is established from the earliest relationship.

Inequality of power exists not only among people, but also between aspects of the individual's mind: just as threats and punishments are inflicted by one person or group over another, so also one part of the self may dominate another. This process is observable in self-destructive beha-viours, whether general depression or specific forms of self-punishment. A depressed adult patient for example bullies himself habitually and com-pulsively, showing me how he hates himself by calling himself 'idiot! worthless fool!'. Even though we both recognise that this pattern comes from his relationship with his abusive father, he continues to destroy his relationships and waste his abilities with his self-loathing. This dynamic expresses itself in the transferential relationship. For example, my patient's determination to stay the same might irritate me, nudging me into becoming something like a bully myself who feels justified in humiliating his victim. If this situation can be translated as the patient's repetition compulsion and the therapist's counter-transference, then it may be worked with constructively.

A psychotherapist working with bullies begins to notice patterns. One example is the bully's characteristic love of rules. These may ultimately add up to the 'banality of evil' (Arendt 1994) but may cast some light on the abuser's frame of mind. For example, Tandy, the torturer from Goole mentioned earlier, showed no interest or regret when it was finally discovered that his victim had in fact not stolen the drugs. Tandy maintained that his unbelievable acts of cruelty were justified because, he claimed, his victim treated him disrespectfully. 'He was asking for it . . . he was taking the piss!' Being treated with disrespect is regarded as the ultimate crime in the subculture of prison. 'You dissing me?' is a common warning. Another example is the boy who said to me, 'No one touches my mum, no one says anything about my mum! Otherwise they'll get it!' He was oblivious to the fact that he had hurt his mother deeply by raping his sister and by pushing his mother to the ground during the row following his sister's disclosure. The bully's blindness to how he has made himself an exception to his rule is partly due to his unconscious need to right a wrong done to him in the past. Someone in his history broke the rules when they abused him. This kind of injustice and grievance can provide an opening in therapy to understand the inner reality of the abuser, that is, the victim in the perpetrator (Cordess & Cox 1996). Through objectively acknowledging his own hurt, the abuser might begin to see how he was trying to right a wrong done to him by inflicting on someone else the abuse that was done to him, rather than face the vulnerability and helplessness he experienced as an abuser's victim. In this way, the bully might begin to understand the meaning of his behaviour and how he has confused himself by taking revenge on an easier target than his original perpetrator.

Psychotherapeutic intervention in the school environment

A psychoanalytic psychotherapist notices how the bullying behaviour within the individual and between individuals is reflected in the ethos of an organisation and the wider society. But how to make that transition from the individual to social reality? A therapist is unlikely to have a remit to enlighten whole organisations. And if attempted, would it not detract from the psychotherapist's proper role to treat individual dysfunction? There are times when it is the system that needs treating rather than an individual.

When this is acknowledged the organisation is halfway to working out the problem. Instead, there is often an endless round of identifying individuals as 'the problem'. But confining the intervention to treating individuals merely classifies and divides them into bully or victim and invites blame. Without also attending to the social system in which the problem exists our work risks being little more than a straw in the wind.

This problem was exemplified in a conference on bullying some years ago at the Anna Freud Centre where psychotherapists presented three treatment cases to an audience of mainly educationalists. There were some observations of the oedipal conflicts that had led these boys to develop insecure identifications with their fathers. Some modest improvement was seen in one boy with bullying behaviour after 'only two and a half years of psychotherapy three times a week'. The audience was understandably dismayed by this apparently small progress from such intensive work. Fortunately, the psychodynamic discussion was balanced by contributions from a head teacher, Michael Marland, who referred to the prevalence of pupils who were afraid of being bullied in his and other schools. He spoke about the strategy developed by himself and colleagues, a tutorial system of constant consultation with pupils. 'A tutor,' he said, 'is a teacher whose subject is the pupils themselves' (Marland 1993: 332). The function of the tutorial group is to concentrate on all aspects of the children's relationships not only problematic behaviours and to encourage them to speak out, make decisions and choose their own strategies. The consultation structure functions as an antidote to the law of the jungle by nurturing a mature and democratic environment and promoting the self-esteem of individuals. Marland reported a decline in bullying incidents over the three-year period since the implementation of the consultation system (Marland 1993).

There is by now a substantial literature on interventions to address bullying in schools, for example, classroom courts, restorative justice, peer mediation (Childline 1996: 107; Kidscape; Rigby 2002: 255–6) or the community approach described in Randall (1996). The first step highlighted by these initiatives is to raise awareness of repeated patterns of bullying behaviour rather than treating separate incidents as isolated events. Group-work interventions for disruptive children in schools have limited effectiveness if attempted in isolation from the wider social context (Canham & Emanuel 2000; Dwivedi 1993; Woods 1996). All these studies draw attention to the need for changes in the staff ethos highlighting ways in which staff exercise control by subtle and not so subtle uses of humiliation (Adams 1992: 70). The curriculum itself can assist teachers to exercise their authority in non-abusive styles. A sea change in the culture needs to permeate the hierarchy: a staff group cannot effectively promote a non-abusive culture if there is intimidation, and injustice within its own structure. Is there a role here for the therapist?

Therapists have to find ways to connect the private space of psycho-therapy to the public sphere of the organisation in order to convey a way of thinking about the violence inherent in bullying from individual to staff to the organisational ethos as a whole. Therapists working in institutions need to engage with the prevailing culture and use whatever influences are available to promote a non-abusive set of norms and expectations both in the handling of students and the functioning of the staff organisation. Openness of communication is the aim. Equality of status is necessarily limited where the maintenance of authority is crucial but equality of rights such as the right to speak out, the right not to be violated, is achievable. A therapist can provide a specialised resource to the staff in drawing attention to these principles and debating them. Sometimes the therapist has to ask uncomfortable questions such as, 'What is the message we are giving students, if we as the staff group behave in certain ways?' Certainly such uncomfortable questions are preferable to the mystification that can sur-round psychodynamic thinking which, at its worst, may be used to excuse anti-social behaviour.

When the family becomes the cradle of violence

Before the social group was the family. Bentovim (1995) condensed many years of experience of working with families with a history of abuse into the concept of the 'trauma organised system'. He found that abuse was inextricably linked with trauma in the family and with the defences erected against re-experiencing the trauma. The function of the family system is to keep the trauma hidden by silencing the victim through processes of blame and disqualification. Through such experiences victims come to blame themselves. For example, the abuser exploits the dependency needs and separation fears of other family members. The victimiser blots out any thoughts, actions or statements that threaten to destabilise the structure that perpetuates the abuse, just as the traumatised individual fends off conscious awareness of a traumatic past that is being expressed in the form of symptoms. The abusive or 'trauma-organised' family creates an imper-meable barrier against the outer world and all discourse is devoted to maintaining its interior stability. Any family member who threatens to disrupt this protection against becoming aware of the trauma faces exclu-sion. The individual carrying the victim experience is punished and silenced with more abuse or rejection if they communicate distress or anger (Bentovim 1995: 47). The family members' unconscious assumptions about each other are powerfully held and communications are constantly turned back on themselves and reinforced. These roles are described by Bentovim as interlocking, since change in one member's behaviour would destabilise the system. Deeply ingrained learning takes place in the children (soon-to-be-adults) who become the products of this sort of environment. Young abusers who come from such trauma organised families identify with this system, which then becomes an organiser of their internal worlds (Woods 2003: 25–30).

Clearly, abuse does not arise as some random, isolated act of aggression but is part of a pattern of an ongoing culture with roots in the family. The child has very limited choices in this situation. Although the roles may fluctuate, there is an obvious dichotomy between those who have power and those without power. The abuser may be ridden with anxiety about disclosures of their abusive behaviour while the apparent victim may hold secret notions of holding power over their abuser in the knowledge of the abuse. There are intricate connections between the power and vulnerability of victim and abuser, two sides, as it were, of the same coin.

When a therapeutic intervention is allowed into the 'trauma organised' family those members who have occupied the role of victim have been treated with so little regard that they are dominated by low self-esteem (Rigby 2002). Aggression in the victim has been suppressed, just as awareness of vulnerability is suppressed in the perpetrator. There is no absolute distinction between victim and bully; in the inner world the one contains the other. A child may choose to become the bully after years of being bullied: the worm turns. One boy clearly remembers the day when he decided that 'no one will ever push me around again' regardless of how much he was hurt in the process. More insight perhaps was shown, eventually, by the bullying father in Strindberg's *Dance of Death* who said, when confronted by the effects of his destructiveness, 'Life was cruel to me so I became cruel' (Strindberg 1899: 96).

The typical problem for the therapist who enters into a dyadic relationship with either chronic victim or abuser is that the patient's bully or victim self will attempt by every means to get the therapist to conform to the complementary role. At its worst, each side of the bully–victim dyad seems chained to its role in a relentless dance of death, in which habitual bullies seems fixed in their disregard of even their own interests, while chronic victims seem unaware of how they have provoked abusive treatment. People beginning treatment are usually not ready to relinquish the part for which they feel predestined. The defensive system is desperately needed, primarily to ward off psychic pain arising from the trauma emanating from the original family experience. A therapist has to negotiate the patient's terror that he might be coerced within the treatment. Countertransference is an especially important source of information as to when these dynamics begin to occur.

In psychotherapeutic treatment, as the fixed nature of these interlocking roles becomes more evident, the other side of the picture painstakingly and painfully enters into consciousness. Whether occupying the role of bully or victim, the opposite is perceived to be unbearable. It remains as it were the dark side of the moon. A powerful barrier exists to protect the bully against the pain of recognising the victim within and to protect the victim against recognising the bully within, but the task of psychoanalytic psychotherapy is to make what was unconscious available to the ego. Bullies who become aware of the victim in themselves are more open to change, like the father in Strindberg's play. Achieving 'victim empathy' is well known by cognitive behavioural therapists as an important step in the completion of treatment for a perpetrator. Equally when victims recover their power and draw on some aggression in the form of assertion of their rights, then they are much less likely to go on being victimised. But interpreting the dynamics between therapist and patient and within the patient's inner world is, in my experience, necessary but rarely sufficient. A third element has to enter in order to prevent therapeutic experience deteriorating into bully/victim dichotomy. This third element is represented by the role of the father.

The role of the father

Direct work with anti-social or violent young males shows the central significance of the role of the father and how the lack of a benign father figure promotes delinquent or anti-social behaviour (Perelberg 1999: 7–8). Children from homes without a father are statistically more likely to be delinquent, and/or self-destructive (Trowell & Etchegoyen 2002: 201). The boy without a father constructs an idealised or denigrated image of the father with which he identifies, thereby attempting to compensate for his lack of paternal nurture that he needs as much as nurturing from his mother. Fathering is often thought about as complementing mothering by standing for limits (Trowell & Etchegoyen 2002: 23). If there are no limits to acceptable behaviour the child's omnipotence produces its own terrors (Trowell & Etchegoyen 2002: 188). The father's 'no' seems to function as a protection against such failures in child development. The father modifies the child's internal world by representing the external world while recognising the impulses and desires of the child. This triangulation in normal development between child, mother and father is thought to be crucial for the development of an individual's capacity to tolerate frustration and think creatively. In Britton's terms: 'The internalisation of the Oedipal triangle creates a mental space' (Britton 2000: 12). This is also linked to a therapeutic principle expounded in the work of Ogden who talks of 'the analytic third', the product of what happens between therapist and patient based on the oedipal configuration. In addition to the I and thou of therapist and patient, there is a third 'intersubjective' element; sometimes it is the world out there, the patient's existence in the world with all its dangers for him, and also the third 'in here', the 'third' that is created between therapist and patient (Ogden 1966: 883–5). The experience of father, as the one who stands between illusory unity with mother is crucial in the relative success with which the infant is able to separate from the mother and to feel himself to be an effective individual.

The therapist can create a triangular space by acknowledging the patient's family or the outside world. For example, in therapy with self-harming young people, the therapist can ask, when the time is right, about the effects on others of their continued self-harm. In other words, who does the self-harmer really want to hurt and why? In the case of perpetrators, there are also significant others as well as the school authority, such as youth justice, or social services, which can be presented as representing a different type of parent to the abusive parent of their family. It may come as a revelation to the young perpetrator from an abusive family when he comes up against limits that are not only firm but fair. When the therapist acknowledges this external reality he frees himself from taking the position of a bullying superego that would have rendered him therapeutically impotent. In group therapy, the third dimension is instantly present in the other group members who will be able to give feedback in ways often unavailable to the therapist. By these and other means it becomes possible to disentangle the roles and provide a therapeutic bridge that avoids being drawn into the repetition of abuse, and the bully/victim dichotomy.

While these notions are intended primarily for work in the consulting room, they may equally well serve therapeutic aims in the social context. By understanding the vital role of a 'third' a school can be helped to focus on the need to create a culture of firm and containing authority. The symbolic parenting provided by a school while nurturing at times, is needed not only to meet the individual's educational needs but also to enable the child to recognise and tolerate limits, separations and losses.

Making psychodynamics relevant to the school

Understanding the victim

Teaching staff are sometimes mystified by the child who regularly seems to be the target of bullying. Randall (1996: 210) quotes research by Olweus in Norway on the 'provocative victim', someone who actively seeks out those who would conform to an abusive parental image. Attachment theory is very helpful in understanding the chronic victim and the invitation they seem to give, albeit unconsciously, to the abuser (DeZulueta 1993: 108). Whether from a management or therapeutic point of view there may be great difficulty in coping with the particular kind of victim who seems to draw out the bully in others. This observation is not about re-allocating blame, because the bully too will be ready to play his part in this perverse kind of attachment. The strength of these perverse attachments may be drawn from the biologically determined bonds between infant and parent. These bonds are understood in attachment theory as a matter of survival, literally of life and death (Bowlby 1969). When a secure attachment based on love and trust cannot be established because the caregiver is an abusive figure, the attachment will be likely to be based on the dominance and submission of bully and victim (DeZulueta 1993).

The psychodynamic perspective gives a more detailed answer to the question as to why habitual victims seek out suffering when they complain so readily about it. Novick and Novick (1998) made an extensive study of masochism and one of their conclusions was that the masochist triumphs because through a masochistic position they acquire a sense of being in control. 'Victory through defeat' is a very real triumph for some who can thereby demonstrate to the world that they have been mistreated, that they should be better served and that they are innocent and morally superior, certainly free of the guilt and the need for punishment now very conveniently located in the other. The payoffs are considerable.

Masochism can also become a survival strategy in some situations, when the victim appears to appease the bully while secretly nurturing a fantasy of being powerful and in control of the bully. David Pelzer has written a horrifying autobiographical account of child abuse: at certain points the abused and apparently powerless child morally triumphs over the mad and out of control adult (Pelzer 1995: 420). A similar phenomenon can be seen in the relatives or partners of some perpetrators who cling to the conviction that they can control a known abuser and limit their activities. There are mothers who protect a paedophile uncle or grandfather in the belief that they can prevent the worst of their behaviour. Maxine Carr, the former girlfriend of the murderer Ian Huntley, was reported to have said that she blames herself for the deaths of the girls of Soham because she should have been there to prevent him from killing them.

Understanding the bully

The bully too is under an unconscious compulsion to repeat distorted and anti-social attachment patterns. But understanding this may not in itself open the way for change. Assessment is clearly of crucial importance. Childline (1996: 111) quotes research (from Olweus in Norway) that shows how the young bully may develop into a criminal in the future. Treatment, at least in the current state of knowledge, may be futile in some cases. Sometimes, the only recourse is to exclude the bully, not only from school, but from society by incarceration, providing temporary relief for others, but little hope of change for him. With young people, however, there may be more chance of effective treatment because of the still unformed nature of their personality and the accessibility of childhood experience for mental processing.

The bully only becomes aware of the victim in himself when he is caught. Therapeutically this is a crucial moment because the bully's tendency is to re-establish the bully/victim dyad. Separating him out as the identified bully is unlikely on its own to produce change, because the sadistic nature of his relationships must be understood and worked through rather than re-enacted. Again the existence of a third element in the treatment facilitates this work. A boy who has perpetrated a crime, for example, needs to become aware that he has disgraced and offended not only the person he assaulted and his family, but also society and its norms: this fact needs to be taken on board. He may be required to attend sessions and reports will have to be written. None of this will be particularly welcome and may seem to him an imposition forced on him. However, it can serve the purpose of focusing the boy's mind on questioning why this fuss is being made by the authorities. This third element, society, and its concern about his offence, creates a more effective space for thinking than a traditionally exclusive one to one. The therapy in this model (Woods 2003) may help him renegotiate his relationship with the social world. And, even more importantly, it is an antidote to the kind of secrecy that in his family would have engendered abuse.

Conclusion

The goal of bullying is not simply to persecute another, but to preserve the power of the bully, which may require the continued survival of the other. This can take the form of breaking the spirit of the victim. A classic depiction of the attachment between torturer and victim is Orwell's *Nineteen Eighty Four*, where Winston is so terrorised that he surrenders his lover: 'Do it to her!' he says. At this point the interrogator has won and Winston has 'learned to love Big Brother' (Orwell 1948: 287). A more recent version is presented in Harold Pinter's *One for the Road*, where the interrogator O'Brien casually kills the child of the political prisoner thus effortlessly proving his 'superiority'. Both sadistic killers demonstrate an adherence to their own set of rules. No matter how half-baked and illogical, each has a system of beliefs, which not only justify the cruelty, but serve some dependency need in the abuser. From the exalted ideal of racial purity, down to the indignation at some imagined slight in the playground, it seems there is a need in the perpetrator for faith in something that preserves him from inner chaos, something like a father figure that will protect and preserve the terrified abuser from what he most dreads; ultimately this may be, at an unconscious level the annihilation by a primitive mother figure (Glasser 1964). It certainly is the case that the vast majority of abusers are male and have disordered relationships with women (Fromm 1973: 548). Therapeutically, this yearning for some kind of father figure to provide safety from trauma may be used to advantage if the former bully himself eventually comes to realise his own needs.

The privilege of the psychotherapist is to see that the aggression is as much to do with the bully's own terrors as that of the victim. In this way a psychotherapist may promote an understanding of the meaning of violence, both in the general sphere and in specific cases; in its ambiguity, aggression may convey both the realisation and the annihilation of the self. Unfortunately, many therapists forget that colleagues in other professions are also combating the same complex forces, albeit in a different way, and sometimes without the knowledge to point in a helpful direction. If we have a contract with an organisation such as a school, we have a duty to make psychodynamics relevant to the tasks of that institution. When therapists are asked to think about the far-reaching effects of human destructiveness they must first consider the relevance of the psychotherapy being practised, because it is all too easy to be drawn into repetitions of abuse and trauma, if only by being ineffective. When therapists are prepared to share their knowledge with colleagues, then they find that the social dimension gives greater meaning to processes seen in the consulting room.

References

Adams, A. (1992) *Bullying at Work*, London: Virago

Arendt, H. (1994) *Eichmann in Jerusalem; A Report on the Banality of Evil*, London: Penguin

Bentovim, A. (1995) *Trauma Organised Systems*, London: Karnac

Bowlby, J. (1969) *Attachment*, London: Penguin

Britton, R. (2000) 'On sharing psychic space', *Bulletin of the Society of Psychoanalytic Marital Psychotherapists* May: 10–16

Canham, H. and Emanuel, L. (2000) 'Tied together feelings: group psychotherapy with latency children', *Journal of Child Psychotherapy* 26: 2

Childline (1996) *Why Me? Children talking to Childline about Bullying*, London: Childline

Cordess, C. and Cox, M. (eds) (1996) *Forensic Psychotherapy; Crime, Psychodynamics and the Offender Patient*, London: Jessica Kingsley

DeZulueta, F. (1993) *From Pain to Violence*, London: Whurr

Dwivedi, K.N. (1993) *Group Work with Children and Adolescents*, London: Jessica Kingsley

Fromm, E. (1973) *The Anatomy of Human Destructiveness*, London: Penguin

Gilligan, J. (1996) *Violence: Reflections on our Deadliest Epidemic*, New York: Puttnams; London: Jessica Kingsley

Glasser, M. (1964) 'Aggression and sadism in the perversions', in *Sexual Deviation*, I. Rosen (ed.), Oxford: Oxford University Press

Golding, W. (1974) *The Lord of the Flies*, London: Penguin

Hill, S. (1970) *I'm the King of the Castle*, London: Penguin

Kidscape Publication, 2 Grosvenor Gardens, London, SW1W 0DH

Marland, M. (1993) 'Bullying; how schools can make a difference', *The Bulletin of the Anna Freud Centre* 16: 4

Novick, J. and Novick, K. (1998) *Fearful Symmetry*, London: Routledge

Ogden, T.H. (1966) 'Reconsidering three aspects of psychoanalytic technique', *International Journal of Psycho-analysis* 77: 883–99

Orwell, G. (1948) *Nineteen Eighty Four*, London: Penguin

Pelzer, D. (1995) *A Child Called It*, London: Orion Press

Perelberg, R.J. (1999) *Psychoanalytic Understanding of Violence and Suicide*, London: Routledge

Randall, P. (1996) *A Community Approach to Bullying*, London: Trentham Books

Rigby, K. (2002) *New Perspectives on Bullying*, London: Jessica Kingsley

Strindberg, A. (1899) 'Dance of Death' in *Collected Plays of August Strindberg*, London: Penguin

Trowell, J. and Etchegoyen, A. (2002) *The Importance of Fathers*, London: Brunner-Routledge

Waddell, M. (2002) 'The psychodynamics of bullying', *Free Associations* 9 2(50): 189–210

Winnicott, D.W. (1962) 'Providing for the child in health and crisis' in *The Maturational Processes and the Facilitating Environment*, London: Hogarth Press

Woods, J. (1986) 'The boundary between psychotherapy and therapeutic teaching' *Journal of Child Psychotherapy* 12: 2

Woods, J. (1996) 'Handling violence in child group therapy', *Group Analysis* 29: 1

Woods, J. (2003) *Boys Who Have Abused*, London: Jessica Kingsley

Chapter 10

On a hiding to nothing? Work with women affected by violence

Rose Christie

Introduction

This chapter explores psychoanalytic work with a particular group of women in whose lives violence has played a significant part. The title reflects a question posed by the nature of self-defeating, destructive solutions employed by the patient group in response to their overwhelming experiences and the formidable challenges of psychoanalytic work in a setting limited by time and frequency. These women were living at or below the poverty line, with minimal education and without previous psychological intervention. Their lives were characterised by high levels of material deprivation, with a real sense of struggle for survival existing alongside, and interacting with, internal deprivation and conflict. They represented one of the most deprived and marginalised groups in 21st century Britain.

The therapeutic work described took place in a community-based organisation offering local women once-weekly sessions for one year as part of a project entitled 'Insight into Violence'. The service was established 20 years ago to provide a professionally staffed psychoanalytic psychotherapy service to women living in a deprived area of inner London.

A particular style of working was developed in response both to the requirements of women dealing with experiences of high levels of aggression and violence and those of the service within which the work takes place. I will highlight the importance of a containing and welcoming environment; the therapist's use of an adaptive style of responding to the patient in order to foster a strong therapeutic alliance; a focus on the here-and-now within the session; the use of analyst-centred interpretations and forging an alliance with the patient's particular strengths.

Understanding female aggression and destructiveness

This setting offers an opportunity to focus on and explore in depth the particular impact on the female psyche of experiences of external and internal aggression. There are features common to these female responses that appear with regularity, each woman with her own unique configurations and adaptations.

The internalised nature of female aggression is a predominant feature. The impact of the maternal relationship on the female infant is crucial. In unfavourable circumstances, the infant's healthy protests at being separated from mother and the developing child's aggressive self-assertive impulses are met by the mother's rejection or retaliation. This sets up a response of turning the expression of the aggressive impulses back on the self in order to secure her relationship with mother on whom she depends for nurturance and protection. The little girl is faced with core complex anxieties (Glasser 1979): abandonment by her mother if she shows her aggressive self-assertion and engulfment by mother if she swallows her self-assertive gestures and hides her separate identity.

The little girl's proclivity to internalise her aggression is reinforced by having a female body like her mother. Perelberg quotes Irigaray's (1989) description of the little girl as having 'the mother, in some sense, in her skin, in the humidity of the mucous membranes, in the intimacy of her most intimate parts, in the mystery of her relation to gestation, birth and to her sexual identity' (1997: 133). Perelberg (1997) describes the female's struggle to separate from her mother and gain a sense of her own identity and body. This process requires an engagement on the part of the mother in a creative, positive use of aggression to cut the ties. Birksted-Breen (1997) and Lawrence (2002), using their work with female anorexic patients, highlight the impact of the failure to separate from a feared, envied but longed for maternal figure. The dynamics of failed separation with subsequent attacks on the body, mind, self and object who might offer sustenance, are also omnipresent features of work with women whose lives have been dominated by violent aggression. Their attachments to and separations from their mothers, are sometimes incomplete and often take the form of a brutal severing of an adhesive, destructive attachment. This leaves the woman as an adult with a catastrophic or failed separation from a maternal object who remains fused in the internal world in the form of a malignant destructive imago. This internal configuration is attacked in the form of aggressive acts on the self. Commonly, the patients present with symptoms of self-neglect (failing to wash, eat, seek help), or active violent and destructive behaviours against the self (cutting, burning, starving). Many women present histories of long-term depressive illness and suicide attempts. The incidence of disease within the body is also prevalent, extreme dysfunction of the female reproductive organs is common.

Lawrence (2002) describes the girl as having, 'an urge to fill her inner world with good objects. This urge contributes to the intensity of the introjective processes, which are reinforced by the receptive nature of her genital, something innately known about by the little girl' (2002: 841). However, the young girl also fears that something dangerous could get inside and damage her. Fears of intrusion, invasion and internal damage thus dominate. The nurturing offered by the maternal figure has the potential to intrude, invade and suffocate and this generates confusion between nourishing and harmful intrusive experience. The image of the female as a passive, receptive object, from the female as the passive recipient of active male sexual intrusions to the familial, societal, religious and cultural ideals that pervade, compound the individual woman's struggle to access and utilise her aggressive aspect.

For those women who are mothers, the struggle to relate to their children provides a further forum within which the internal conflicts around their own aggression and potential for violent behaviour are played out. In female perversion, the infant becomes the mother's narcissistic object. The intrusive potential of the primary relationship may be exploited by the mother who uses her daughter to contain her own overwhelming feelings of aggression, fear and hatred. Many women reported their longing for a child (especially a daughter) so that they would have someone to love them or do the things that they could not. It is painfully clear that these are expressions of the mother's own need for mirroring, containment and a safe connection with another who exists primarily to provide for her own infantile needs. These women typically present resistance and often paranoid fears for the child (a projection of their own aggressive impulses) at points of their child's natural separation from them: birth, weaning, toddlerhood and school. In the transference, intrusive projection and projective identification are often extremely intense. For example, in the case of the woman I describe later, this took the form of a mix of terror (of the internal and external aggressor), despair and an intense longing to enfold, indeed to take in and therefore annihilate, the other. Carvalho (2002) has used the term 'occupation of the object', which accurately describes the aggressive psychic intrusion into the other experienced in the transference and originally by the infant.

These mothers struggle on a conscious level to protect and nurture their children but have few inner resources from which to draw for this demanding task. The patients' material suggests that many of these mothers use their infants as a fetish or transitional object to gain relief from sexual tension and anxiety (Welldon 1988a). For many of these women the father was absent, indifferent, violent or abusive. This scene was compounded by the attitude of the mother perpetuating the image of the father as brutal or useless. Indeed, most of the women have a deeply entrenched internal fear of the male who is perceived as all-powerful alongside their own overwhelming vulnerability. Denigration is often employed in an attempt to defend against the overwhelming fear of this power, oscillating with longing for the protection of the idealised powerful male figure. I would add that the mothers use their infants to contain their own unprocessed aggressive impulses. Our observations bear out Lloyd-Owen's description:

> [P]erverse women do not in the main turn to outsiders to try to master or communicate their own earlier abuse. They use the whole of their own bodies and their babies for this purpose. What goes into or comes out of their bodies is used not to express love but hate or revenge. What should be creative becomes perverse.
>
> (2003: 295)

Welldon (1988a, 2001) speaks of transgenerational patterns of perverse responses of mothers to their children a pattern frequently observed in this population of women served by the centre. She highlights elements of retaliation by the female against her own mother in the destructive relationship with her infant (1988a: 16). The service's crèche provides an opportunity to observe the interactions between the mothers and their young children. Frequently the mother makes demands on their child as though they were an adult. The mother sometimes accuses her infant of malicious behaviours towards them as if the infant is consciously choosing to persecute her. Parker specifically links separation difficulties with the mother's need for the child as her self-object. In order to facilitate separation, she must relinquish the child from her own sphere, acknowledging its own separate reality. When mother cannot accept her ambivalent feelings, or if her hatred predominates and remains unconscious, then separation is problematic:

> Only via 'destroying' her baby can she be said to have achieved the use of an infant, meaning a relationship to the baby as a person increasingly separate from herself. For this destruction to remain benign and non-retaliatory – for the baby to survive – the mother's progress to object usage in relation to the baby needs to be accompanied by love. Once again we see the pivotal importance of a mother achieving a recognition of her ambivalence.
>
> (Parker 1995: 116)

In the work with these women the presence of their own mother is pervasive as evident in the frequent examples of psychosomatic linkage between mothers and their children (McDougall 1989). The image of the all-providing maternal presence, with whom there is only blissful union and no separation, remains a powerful fantasy for many of these patients. This operates alongside a reality of neglect and abandonment, often accompanied by clinging, intrusive, physically or sexually violent mothering. In this context, the concept of the core complex (Glasser 1979) is apposite. Mounting aggressive feelings, linked with intense conflicts aroused by the infant's dependence and need for union with the mother, alongside the compulsion to destroy the engulfing, intrusive mother, is a dynamic observable within the transference and the patients' descriptions of their emotional lives. Sexualisation of these murderous feelings towards the engulfing object provides another solution to the dilemma of wanting to destroy the needed object. The presence of a maternal eroticised transference is a common feature within this work.

When confronted with the primitive internal landscapes presented by these patients, full of persecuting, terrorising objects, I often feel that the subject is a kind of offering or 'sacrificial lamb', permanently attempting to placate or make a truce with furious, vengeful internal gods. Perhaps this echoes the experience of the infants in the crèche and the early experiences of the patients themselves.

Working with female aggression and destructiveness

In what would generally be thought of as short- or medium-term work one of the most important questions to address is what can we offer in this setting? How can we work with deeply disturbed patients within their life context of few resources and little acknowledgement of their existence or needs?

The meaning of the setting

The meaning of the analytic setting brings the important function of the father into focus. The pivotal role of the father is crucial in developmental terms facilitating the process of separation from mother and representing a real and symbolic third element in the internal and external world of the child. Target and Fonagy (2002) write of the special vulnerability of children with absent or unavailable fathers and the profound impact of this on the processes of separation from the primary object:

> The father is necessary to support the child's aggressive drives and to help him mourn the loss of the earlier phase-specific relationship to the mother. The importance of this function is highlighted in cases where the mother is over-invested in the child, who may be forced to carry the burden of the mother's own sexual and aggressive conflicts.
>
> (2002: 49)

For the patient entering a therapeutic environment the setting itself provides the possibility of an experience of triangulation. The setting can ameliorate the development of an all-consuming dyad between patient and analyst. As Perelberg describes: 'The analytic setting itself, [which] is experienced as a symbolic system that stands for the father and thus mediates in the phantasies of fusion with the mother' (Perelberg 1999: 8).

In this particular setting the female therapists and the service offered both perform the function of the potential father figure. The importance of boundaries, and the imposition of these, the abstinent but attentive analytic stance and the leading of the patient into the area of language, the area of symbolic functioning, all contribute to presenting patients with a valuing and respectful attitude to masculine aspects. Chasseguet-Smirgel writes: 'If the imago of the mother as holder of the paternal penis dominates, the triangular situation begins in outline' (1970: 117).

One of the first challenges facing this group of patients is to simply tolerate being noticed and offered something. The project's building immediately offers them the possibility of a positive transference: although old and rundown, formerly a Victorian workhouse, it is a massive construction conveying a solid, reliable object. Many women arrive early for their sessions, perhaps leaving their children in the crèche and retiring to the quiet waiting room, where they sit in private reflection. One patient contrasted this with her home environment as a single parent with five children under the age of 10 in a three-bedroom flat. Beyond accepting a place of relative peace in the midst of a noisy intrusive and disruptive life, I sense that this environment generates in these patients an unconscious longing for the presence of a 'third' and the potential for containment and mediation. These patients are accustomed to a persecuting and neglectful environment. Consequently, their responses to offers of any kind, especially one involving an intimate relationship, are characterised by suspicion and fear. The institution represents the possibility of a secure and containing object which notices their needs and treats them with respect (Welldon 1988b).

The term 'the brick mother' has been adopted by the project's staff from patients' feedback about their initial contact with the place. This eloquently describes their transference to a solid object offering a combination of firmness and something positively maternal. The presence of the institution as a third object offers patients the opportunity to face the challenge of separating from mother allowing the presence of a paternal, non-retaliatory presence to mediate the more intense archetypal maternal imagos. The centre staffed by women offers the patients a model of the positive and creative use of aggression by females in a patriarchal culture where traditionally aggression in females has been discouraged.

Assessment

In the manner of a child with a new object in an unfamiliar setting, I have observed new patients cautiously approaching, senses at breaking point, extremely watchful, sometimes followed by turning the experience over and over, sometimes daring to metaphorically touch, but often keeping their distance. This has close associations to the states of hyper-arousal present in post-traumatic states (Taylor 1998).

Interpreting this display of caution in relation to past experiences of abuse and trauma at assessment seems to allow some patients to engage with the therapeutic process. For some this direct acknowledgement brings forth a torrent of grief. Others respond by attacking themselves: 'I should be able to cope better, I have always been useless, the world would be a better place if I were dead.' Expressions of anger towards an external object are rare: the local services are an exception as their attempts to provide housing, healthcare and social support are almost universally experienced as inadequate, harsh and damaging. This is the first evidence of protest towards an object that, lacking a human face and distant enough, may be attacked in relative safety.

When the realities of the external world are characterised by extremes of hardship and uncertainty the challenges of relating to an internal world that is also infused with persecutory experience are heightened. In response to this the service has developed a framework of thinking that includes an emphasis on the importance of recognising the real vicissitudes of the patients' lives within the work itself. This acknowledgement of the real impact of hardship in the external world seems to make the painful process of exploring the internal world more bearable.

The underlying, previously unexplored experiences of abandonment and trauma are often revealed at assessment. This raises technical questions about opening traumatised areas of the inner world within a relatively short timeframe. How much can be explored, in what depth, within this setting? From this challenge a way of working has developed that simply offers each new patient the opportunity to explore her external and internal worlds. All patients have some desire for understanding, either to understand themselves, or to be understood by another (Steiner 1993).

It is interesting to note that several women who approached the service initially and failed to engage with the process, re-referred themselves some time later and proceeded into the work. This, I think reflects the therapist's manifest trust and respect for the patient's ability to intuitively choose the appropriate timing of the intervention. For others, the offer is overwhelming and they intuitively reject the offer of a containing space. We can only speculate about the underlying anxieties evoked, but the prospect of exposing the traumatised inner self, with inadequate time to process the experience, is likely to deter some patients from engaging. The balance between the fear of letting go the defences originally created to avoid psychic destruction versus the longing for some more bearable state, involving relating differently to the self, others and the environment, poses a terrible dilemma for the patient (McDougall 1989). In a real sense, each patient is invited to make a choice and her choice is respected. The decision to reject treatment can take place at the point of referral, assessment or when a contract is offered. Most women who choose to begin ongoing sessions stay for the whole term of their contract.

I think that patients who choose to engage with the process know what they are exposing themselves to at some level. They are part of a group capable of contemplating internal movement as if there is a space inside in which something can happen. This may be equivalent to the child who takes the hand offered by a teacher even though other adults have abused her, in contrast to the child who turns away. The women who can bear to engage may be more able to tolerate their aggressive impulses than those who choose to remain isolated. Something in the act of taking hold can be akin to actively aggressive acts, like squeezing the hand. In this work, I often experience myself in the transference as an object required to invite a kind of safe play fighting, with a balance of active, feisty interaction and concern between the participants.

Adaptive ways of working

Clearly, within this brief timeframe we are aiming for small shifts rather than major breakthroughs. The question 'how much is enough?' is always part of the work and all the more pertinent for mirroring so closely the patient's actual experience of limited resources.

As adults this patient group have experienced ongoing deprivation. In addition, their early experiences are a coagulation of ongoing abuse and neglect. Good aspects of their past and present experiences are difficult to identify. Over 50 percent of patients referred to the project have suffered sexual abuse during childhood and almost all have witnessed, and/or been subjected to, extreme ongoing violence within their family environment. Some women have been taken into local authority care as a consequence of abuses within their homes. Most patients have little or no positive experience of a male presence in their early lives: fathers are either absent or abusive and violent. The quality of mothering received varies but is generally characterised by high levels of neglect, often accompanied by mental health problems.

The patients who present to this project confirm the psychoanalytic idea that females typically react to deprivation by attacking the self rather than the object (Chasseguet-Smirgel 1970; McDougall 1989; Welldon 1988a). Levels of depressive illness are high, as are somatic presentations, all of which can be thought of as enactments of aggressive impulses that cannot be processed, expressed or tolerated mentally. Despite their defensive efforts to preserve the self and consciousness from awareness of terrifying levels of internal destructive aggression, most patients are terrified of the destructive thoughts, feelings or actions they are, or could be, capable of. Many express intense feelings of self-hatred and longing to end their existence, in some form or other saying 'rid me of this monster which is myself'. One possible aim of treatment is to understand that the monster (which is an aspect of the self) needs recognition, a voice and a bearable place within the self.

> One young woman admitted that somewhere she was angry but her feelings were terrifying, like a caged wild animal who would savage anyone who came near; 'You wouldn't want to know what comes into

my head sometimes.' My response, that maybe she thought it better if I did not know, elicited a direct link to her mother who responded to her expressions of need as an attack and violently turned on the child.

Another woman presenting problems with her uncontrollably aggressive adolescent son, described her potential fury as the part of her that would want to smash up everything in sight, including me. Later she admitted that she envied her son because his attacks had been noticed, taken seriously and attended to at school. My interpretation, that she might be asking me to notice an unknown and unrecognised part of her, possibly her forbidden aggressive impulses, provided her with a sense that the unthinkable could be thought about.

Concepts such as the 'good-enough mother' (Winnicott 1965) and 'container-contained' (Bion 1962), describe the mother/therapist's function of accepting, containing, metabolising the chaotic, unbearable, raw sensations presented by these traumatised patients and reintroducing them in a bearable form.

Recognising and valuing the real relationship and fostering the working alliance with the patient's non-neurotic, reasonable aspects alongside the transference relationship, provides the key thinking behind this time-limited work. We attempt to identify and nurture the relatively healthy aspects of each patient in the hope that they will be able to recognise and utilise these to strengthen the ego. These techniques are described by Greenson and Wexler (1969), who stress the analyst's concern and respect for the patient in both their healthy and unhealthy aspects, alongside the pursuit of insight, as the factors that contribute to a good working alliance between patient and therapist. It is important to use procedures, which strengthen the ego functions for gaining understanding: 'A good example is abreaction, which allows the patient to discharge intense emotion and thus, indirectly, makes the ego available for insight' (Greenson & Wexler 1969: 29). Further, allying with healthy aspects of the self is required to modify attacks against the self. In working with violence the therapeutic alliance also serves to allow moderate attacks on the therapist, rendering such attacks safe and survivable.

The transference is typically characterised by intense oscillations between idealisation and denigration, as one would expect when working with this level of disturbance. Much of the work is a demand to contain, continue to think and maintain a stance of neutral availability. Interpretations generally take the form of feeding back and making sense of the unbearable emotions being expressed, often of abandonment, or of being misused by another:

One woman, in her late 50s, after a lifetime of violent relationships and later isolation in an attempt to protect herself and others from her rage, expressed her fury in random verbal attacks, both within and outside of the therapy. I tolerated her attacks in a non-retaliatory manner. When I verbalised her underlying infantile feelings of abandonment, shame, and self-hatred, conveyed over a period in the counter-transference, she curled into a foetal ball, sobbing and sucking her fingers. Later in the work she began to care for herself by joining a literacy class and made reparation by caring for her granddaughter in a loving manner.

The use of primarily analyst-centred interpretations, such as, 'you are afraid that I . . .', or 'It was painful for you when I said . . .' seem to convey a sense of being understood by the therapist, allowing some very anxious patients to stay who would be unable to tolerate a more patient-centred approach: 'Thus one hopes to re-establish oneself as a container . . . or as parents who can think together' (Lloyd-Owen 2003: 294).

The limited timeframe of one year comes into the work from the outset. Perhaps one unconscious factor influencing the patient's choice to engage or not is their capacity to bear this knowledge from the beginning and allow engagement to happen nevertheless, suggesting a latent awareness of a need for attachment, nourishment, separation and loss. The inevitable ending is often denied during the work but some potential ability to rage against the dying of the light is likely to be a prerequisite for beginning. This capacity to rage is a positive aspect of aggression: the ability to register pain and express the complex mix of emotional responses to being hurt, including the wish to defend the vulnerable self by attacking the damaging object.

The impact of the work on the therapist

Working with women who bring enormous levels of need and intense experiences of trauma into their therapy places great demands on the therapist and indeed the service. The therapist needs a well-developed knowledge of her own potential for violence without fearing it. In the daily experience of the work intense counter-transference experiences of terror, physical paralysis, dissociative-type states, hatred, powerlessness, fury, despair, dread, among others, are common. These require much processing, both within and between sessions. The whole team is often called on in unconscious ways to assist this process and regular team process meetings are essential to maintain relatively healthy working relationships. Time for thinking and reflection is an important part of the working space in addition to regular supervision.

Case study

D is a 30-year-old Kurdish woman from Turkey. She had been living in the UK for about 10 years. D was married, aged 15, to a man 10 years older than herself. They had a son and a daughter. D had separated from her husband shortly before her GP referred her to the service. She spoke little English but declined an opportunity to work with a Turkish-speaking counsellor, insisting that she could not speak of her experiences to someone from her own culture. The referral included the information that D was attending the surgery regularly, had a long history of physical complaints, had been intermittently in the care of the local community mental health team and had developed an erotic attachment to one of the male GPs in the practice. There was an underlying appeal to take this difficult and demanding patient off their hands.

My initial impressions included a strong eroticised maternal counter-transference. D conveyed a potent mixture of fear, danger, threat, excitement and curiosity behind her almost lifeless, dishevelled, half-asleep exterior. During the early part of our work, D arrived very early and curled up on a hard bench in the waiting room, like a tramp in the park. Sometimes she slept, but she always made eye contact when I appeared and gathered her belongings to shuffle along to the consulting room. The early work, with its challenges to find any common ground could only be approached in a very intuitive manner. We slowly began to create this space, as much hers as mine. Since the usual means of communication were limited, greater than usual attention was required to what could be termed 'state', which has been described by Albrecht-Schwaber quoting Sander (1995) as:

'[W]holeness in the living system', a 'wholeness of the brain' and of the organism, constructed in continuing process, by the 'complexity of unending interactions, transactions, and exchanges'.

(Albrecht-Schwaber 1998: 668)

These interactions were conveyed non-verbally and mirrored D's need for accurate 'affect attunement' (Stern 1998).

How were we to communicate without shared language? Gestures, facial expressions, body movements, tone of voice became more important than the words spoken. In the first session, I said to D that my lack of Turkish was as much a difficulty as her lack of English. At this she smiled, relieved to find she was not a big problem. This seemed to evoke a powerful early mother/infant scene. I understood this as heralding a healthy part of her seeking a suitable environment in which to explore and describe her experience. Antinucci-Mark suggests that: 'The analyst is the language giving mother . . . The process of the creation of this language is similar to the unfolding of the dynamics between the baby learning how to speak and his mother' (1990: 377). She stresses the creative, playful space within which this process unfolds. My feeling was that D was demanding this of me in our earliest interactions.

It was important to consider D's explicit request for treatment with a therapist who did not speak her mother tongue. She explained that she could not imagine any Turkish therapist tolerating her because she had to talk about things that would be unacceptable within her own culture. I saw in this a condensed description of her experience of rejection by her mother and the shameful feelings this cast on D. She protected her shameful self from re-exposure to possible rejection by translating her experience into another language within the context of a different culture.

My accurate attunement to D's 'state' and sensitivity to her non-verbal communications helped to establish a strong therapeutic alliance. Once she felt I was available to listen, D was eager to tell her story and a lively individual quickly emerged. She found the level of her own aggression a problem partly due to the traditional unacceptability of aggression in women in general and particularly within D's culture. Paradoxically, D approached a women's service, seeking help with what may have been previously regarded as a masculine aspect, her aggressive instinct and its expression within her body and her relationships. D attacked her body with severe somatic defences focused on her female reproductive system and also in her self-neglect, cutting herself and three previous suicide attempts. Her relationships with others had become infused with eroticised feelings and violent outbursts, expressed in occasional physical attacks on her husband and extremely ambivalent relationships with her two children.

D conveyed her history with much affect. She was the second to eldest girl in a family of eight siblings from a small Kurdish village in eastern Turkey. From an early age D became the domestic family slave. Rarely attending school, she spent her time caring for her younger siblings and doing housework. Even this, she felt, was devalued from overhearing her mother telling a neighbour how useless D was at getting the washing clean. At this point, D defiantly stated that another village woman had said, 'she is too young to carry those heavy weights'. My comments (emphasising her positive attributes) about the cleaning she was doing for the family (dealing with the shit and semen on the sheets) were initially met with interest but bemusement. However, this turned to a recognition of something that made sense to her when she said that I was helping her to clean up the sheets, indicating her sense of me allying with her healthy aspect. At this point, she sat back in her chair, looking into the middle distance; I had an image of linen on the line flapping in the wind.

Bion (1959) described the impact of early failures of containment and the impact of this on the ability to learn or pursue profitable relations with any object. D said that when she did go to school 'it was hopeless' because her head was filled with other stuff leaving no space to think or learn. Her mind was occupied by the violent arguments between her parents, and her exposure to violent sexual acts between her parents. This offered us a picture of no space, no thinking and of a violent sado-masochistic parental intercourse, which D recreated within her own marriage.

D knew, at a profound level, that she had embodied the monstrous acts she had witnessed and been subjected to. She responded by self-punishment. Her body had become a container for vile, putrid aggressive impulses. From adolescence D experienced regular urinary infections and she graphically described the green stinking pus which emerged from her passages. The infections swarmed about her lower organs and she had many investigative operations on her uterus and ovaries. She understood this situation as a result of frequent incidents of anal and vaginal rape to which her husband had subjected her. When I suggested that her body could be expressing something of her feelings this made complete sense to her. She said: 'Yes, I cannot say it in words, the smell and the hot pain is like it feels inside me.'

D described a relatively close relationship with her father, despite regular beatings, but he was absent from the family for long periods working abroad. D's relationship with her mother felt totally toxic. Later in our year together the presence of a kinder figure in the shape of her paternal grandmother appeared. D also seemed to find some comfort in relating with her wider childhood environment. The village and its surrounding mountains, the children with whom she played and a sense of cultural belonging were described positively. D had been able to form a positive alliance to those elements in her life that she had experienced as nurturing, as she was able to form a therapeutic alliance within the treatment.

As our work progressed, D became increasingly able to rely on her strong initial positive transference to allow herself to explore the painful and terrifying aspects of her internal world. She tolerated the week-long gaps between sessions relatively well, but would sometimes numb her loneliness with alcohol. After our first short break she missed her session and sheepishly admitted that she hated me for going away. She began to think of her drinking as a way of punishing me for leaving her, destroying her thinking and our achievements. The therapeutic alliance had begun to create a space within which she felt increasingly able to risk attacking the object, me, confident that I would survive, as would the link between us.

Gradually the intensity of D's aggressive, destructive hatred became apparent. She was able to speak of her private fantasy world wherein she took revenge on all those who had hurt her. This included a particular fantasy of castrating her husband and consuming his penis in a tasty stew. Using the adaptive technique of affirming and mirroring her positive aspects, I responded to this material not with a deep interpretation of penis envy or the need to acquire the penetrating aggressive aspects of the male abuser but with a simple affirmation that she was able to think and speak about this act rather than do it. D took this and similar responses, I think as confirmation that her aggressive feelings were tolerable, even understandable and she began to value her ability to creatively discharge them safely. It was around this time that she came to a session and proudly told me that she was going to write down her story in a special book. This indicated identification with myself in the transference, as a positive, thinking object which she was utilising as a model for her own growing ability to think and create. I responded by saying that I thought she was now able to value her own experience and see it as worthy of a special place which she, herself could make. Her physical symptoms lessened and she looked well. In the summer break, D took her children to Turkey to stay by the sea with her sister.

Eight weeks before the end of our contract, with much of the work focusing on our ending, D brought a dream. In the dream, she was a child in her home village. She described how she felt at home, she belonged and was free to play in the mountains. In her wanderings, she met an old wise woman of the village. The woman walked with her and they spoke together of many things. The woman showed her how to make a sacrifice. D was given a young bull calf and was shown how to slit its throat and let the blood flow. This was a rather wonderful, graphic description of an act of creative aggression. Later, the sacrificial animal was roasted and the entire village shared the feast. D told me that the animal was the best of its kind and her offering was received with great solemnity and appreciation. She felt that this dream told her that she was beginning to feel worthy of her place in the world, a good Muslim woman. D explained the wise woman figure as a combination of her grandmother, a mythic wise woman remembered from childhood stories, and myself.

Inevitably the ending after one year's work was experienced as harsh, rigid and punishing. But D could now express these feelings. I also felt her longing to trash the container of the time boundary and preserve the mutual nourishment of the mother–infant symbiosis. Once again, the essential function of the third object in encouraging the dissolution of the dyadic relationship was required, this function being performed by colleagues and within supervision. In her written feedback, which all clients are invited to offer, D wrote: 'I was a baby who could not even crawl, but now I am like a child. I can walk and nearly run.' I think that this expresses the limits of the work (not yet able to run) alongside the progression and crucially, the sense of pride in herself, which she took away from the experience.

References

Albrecht-Schwaber, E. (1998) 'The non-verbal dimension in psychoanalysis: "state" and its clinical vicissitudes', *International Journal of Psycho-Analysis* 79: 667–79

Antinucci-Mark, G. (1990) 'Speaking in tongues in the consulting room or the dialectic of foreignness', *British Journal of Psychotherapy* 6(4): 375–83

Bion, W.R. (1959) 'Attacks on linking', *International Journal of Psycho-Analysis* 40: 308–15

—— (1962) *Learning from Experience*, London: Heinemann

Birksted-Breen, D. (1997) 'Working with an anorexic patient' in *Female Experience: Three Generations of British Women Psychoanalysts on Work with Women*, J. Raphael-Leff and R.J. Perelberg (eds), London and New York: Routledge

Carvalho, R. (2002) 'Psychic retreats revisited: binding primitive destructiveness or securing the object? A matter of emphasis?', *British Journal of Psychotherapy* 19(2): 153–71

Chasseguet-Smirgel, J. (1970) *Female Sexuality: New Psychoanalytic Views*, London: Karnac

Glasser, M. (1979) 'Some aspects of the role of aggression in the perversions' in *Sexual Deviation*, I. Rosen (ed.), Oxford: Oxford University Press

Greenson, R.R. and Wexler, M. (1969) 'The non-transference relationship in the psychoanalytic situation', *International Journal of Psycho-Analysis* 50: 27–39

Irigaray, L. (1989) 'The gesture in psychoanalysis' in *Between Feminism and Psychoanalysis*, T. Breman (ed.), London: Routledge

Lawrence, M. (2002) 'Body, mother, mind. Anorexia, femininity and the intrusive object', *International Journal of Psycho-Analysis* 83: 837–47

Lloyd-Owen, D. (2003) 'Perverse females: their unique psychopathology', *British Journal of Psychotherapy* 19(4): 285–96

McDougall, J. (1989) *Theatres of the Body: A Psychoanalytical Approach to Psychosomatic Illness*, London: Free Association Books

Parker, R. (1995) *Torn in Two. The Experience of Maternal Ambivalence*, London: Virago

Perelberg, R.J. (1997) 'Introduction to Part 1' in *Female Experience: Three Generations of British Women Psychoanalysts on Work with Women*, J. Raphael-Leff and R.J. Perelberg (eds), London and New York: Routledge

—— (1999) 'Introduction' in *Psychoanalytic Understanding of Violence and Suicide*, London: Routledge

Sander, L.W. (1995) 'Thinking about developmental process: Wholeness, specificity, and the organization of conscious experiencing'. Presentation at meeting of American Psychological Association, Div. 39, Santa Monica

Steiner, J. (1993) *Psychic Retreats: Pathological Organisations in Psychotic, Neurotic and Borderline Patients*, London: Routledge

Stern, D.N. (1998) *The Interpersonal World of the Infant*, London: Karnac

Target, M. and Fonagy, P. (2002) 'Fathers in modern psychoanalysis and in society: the role of the father and child development' in *The Importance of Fathers: A Psychoanalytic Re-evaluation*, J. Trowell and A. Etchegoyen (eds.), Hove: Brunner-Routledge

Taylor, D. (1998) 'The psychodynamic assessment of post-traumatic states' in *Understanding Trauma: A Psychoanalytical Approach*, C. Garland (ed.), London: Karnac

Welldon, E.V. (1988a) *Mother, Madonna, Whore*, London: The Guilford Press

—— (1988b) 'Forensic psychotherapy: the practical approach' in *A Practical Guide to Forensic Psychotherapy*, E.V. Welldon and C. Van Velson (eds), London and Bristol, PA: Jessica Kingsley

—— (2001) 'Babies as transitional objects' in *Forensic Psychotherapy and Psychopathology Winnicottian Perspectives*, B. Kahr (ed.), London: Karnac

Winnicott, D.W. (1965) *The Maturational Processes and the Facilitating Environment*, London: Hogarth Press

Chapter 11

Some reflections on the connections between aggression and depression

Leon Kleimberg

Introduction

In his book *The Power and the Glory*, Graham Greene describes the violent war between the Catholic Church and the Mexican government of Cardenas in 1938. He suggests that 'the emergence of hatred is purely the result of a failure of the imagination' (1940: 152). Creativity and imagination, I believe, are closely connected to each other. In fact, I have argued that in some senses psychopathology as a whole can be understood as the failure of the individual to use creativity for living (Kleimberg 2003).

A survey of the literature on depression reveals a variety of views on the different types of depression or depressive experience. Depression can be seen as aggression that is felt towards the object and then turned against the self (Abraham 1924); a failure in the process of mourning (Freud 1917); a healing mechanism (Winnicott 1954); the failure to gratify oral needs (Fenichel 1946); a failure to successfully resolve the depressive position (Klein 1952); or the mother and baby's failure to engage successfully resulting in a narcissistic inflated version of self and other that works as a cover up for such a failure (Rosenfeld 1964).

In this chapter, depression is viewed as aggression attendant on the loss of an object or a psychic loss (Freud 1917). The healthy and creative depression following a loss takes the individual to further progress, enabling them to mourn the loss, come to terms with it, let it go and make the most of what they have. Thus loss may promote development in the inner world and help the individual to use their aggression to transform their internal and external world into opportunities to live, learn and communicate with others (Stewart 1992).

In pathological depression, the internal objects or superego blame the ego for the loss and attack and persecute the ego in a cruel and sadistic way, rather than supporting and comforting the self. When this happens the ego of the individual reacts with submissiveness, loss of self-esteem and depression. In destructive depression, aggression is used to destroy and attack the self or anything or anyone that attempts to intervene in the pathological depressive sado-masochistic status quo created by the individual in order to survive such attacks. Interestingly, it has also been noted that in some circumstances the suffering brought by this depressive sado-masochistic psychic choice not only prevents separateness and growth, but also becomes a source of perverse pleasure in itself (Fenichel 1946).

The capacity to express and transform conscious and unconscious aggression in all of us depends on the development of the symbolic function. Concrete symbolisation is clearly at the root of pathological mourning and therefore of pathology in general. People who are unable to symbolise do not have the creative resources and imagination to transform aggression into a life-giving force (Kleimberg 2003). Some personalities remain undeveloped emotionally and intellectually, unable to separate from their primal objects, incapable of operating in the world of symbols and metaphors: they seem unable to develop beyond a limited level of psychic development and primitive, unimaginative ways of operating (Segal 1991). Unable to progress in their psychic development they cannot mourn their losses or work through separations or endings. These personalities have not developed an adequate symbolic function that could allow primitive aggression to be transformed into life-giving forces conducive to separateness, growth and concern for other people. Without the capacity to use symbols to express aggression, emotions acquire a direct and dangerous concrete reality. Without the capacity to symbolise the individual cannot recover from the loss of the object or protect the object from aggressiveness. These individuals have a very limited capacity to tolerate frustration and most of their life is organised to avoid psychic suffering even if that entails using violent or ruthless means.

In this chapter, I am going to explore a particular type of sado-masochistic pathological depression that I found in Gloria, a patient of mine. As I began to work with Gloria, I was struck by a noticeable absence of imagination and creativity in her presentations of herself and also by a clear connection between this lack of creativity and imagination and the constant hateful, angry and depressive states of mind she lived in. Gloria seemed to lack the psychic resources necessary to use imagination as a means to metabolise her internal and external experience and change her frustrating, painful, hateful and angry life, into a more fruitful, happy and creative one. Her first five years of analysis were a continuous struggle to discover and to understand the absence of her creative resources.

Gloria

Gloria was 39 years old when she started analysis, suffering from severe depression and anxious agitation. In the preliminary interviews to the analysis, it became clear to both of us that she was lost and not really knowing who she was. From the beginning of the analysis Gloria presented a severe depression, a narcissistic personality and intense over-controlled emotionally violent responses that presented as immovable character solutions to emotional conflict. Her emotional responses lacked any creative or imaginative resolution.

Gloria's responses to analytic contacts with me were tense, compliant or submissive. Working with these defensive character traits allowed us to discover the concrete and anxious way she was experiencing me and the analytic process and relationship. Somehow she felt constantly attacked and criticised by me and my interpretations, reacting with silent implosive anger, which she showed me in the next session by presenting herself in a depressed and confused state of mind. Gloria's reactions, when she experienced me as critical of her, had a flat and concrete quality to them. In my counter-transference responses, I had a vivid sense that in Gloria's emotional implosions there was something missing from the analytic process. I became aware that, with Gloria, there was no freedom in our interactions, there was no imagination and there was no sense of relief or liberation as other patients might experience when feeling understood and contained. It began to occur to me that there was some kind of link between Gloria's lack of imagination and her angry emotional reactions and her depression. Gloria's violent emotional responses and concrete experiencing of me made me realise that her lack of imagination was indicative of the absence in some degree of a symbolic function (Segal 1991) that would have allowed Gloria to feel understood in our therapeutic relationship. I soon began to discover that Gloria's inner world was dominated by a highly critical superego. Her critical inner world restricted her capacity to symbolise or sublimate and, in turn, led her to experience me in the analysis as a highly critical analyst who inhibited her capacity to imagine, symbolise or have any kind of inner freedom.

Gloria's background gives some clues as to the origins of her critical inner world. She was the older of two girls from a South American family. Their highly domineering and possessive mother treated the world outside the family as the enemy and convinced her daughters that they were only safe when in her lap. Father was an almost non-existent presence except to placate mother and avoid conflict.

When Gloria came to see me she was very depressed, bulimic and highly involved in shoplifting. Her presenting problem was her inability to live a meaningful life. Her life continued to revolve around her mother back in South America even though she had been living in England for several years. Mother was still ruling her life from 8000 miles away over the telephone and via the post. For example, she would send Gloria weekly parcels of cooked food and other goods ostensibly to keep my patient properly nourished! Gloria would not understand what was so inappropriate about this, except to notice that she felt panicky and suffocated every time the postman rang the doorbell to deliver the parcel or every time she phoned her mother to say thank you for the food! During this period, Gloria would have short dreams of 'twins being killed by a woman'. Given the devastating effect that my comments had on her, the analysis at this stage was almost a non-verbal process. She would feel attacked and criticised by my interpretations or she would feel that I was attacking her 'beloved parents'. She used to describe this period as if she 'did not have an unconscious' nor did she remember her childhood or past history.

The structure of Gloria's critical inner world

The connection between Gloria's aggression and the development of her depression is through the narcissistic defence she established against the pain of separation and the inevitable frustration and loss involved. Every time she tried to separate from her internal or external mother she would encounter fierce attacks from the mother or intense guilt feelings coming from the attacks from her internal superego. She would experience this as being crushed by criticisms or feeling such despair that she wanted to die. As Freud described, 'this super-ego can confront the ego and treat it like an object; and it often treats it very harshly' (1926: 223).

To avoid these critical attacks, Gloria avoided separating from her superego (Rosenfeld 1964). Instead, she chose to merge with it by splitting herself in two parts: a part of her through identification became like the mother and another part of her became the constant victim of attacks inflicted by the part of her that identified with her harsh maternal aspect enshrined in her superego. In consequence she developed a masochistic depression (Abraham 1911; Fenichel 1946) whereby the ego, in order to survive the sadistic attacks of the superego (auditory criticisms, guilt, loss of self-esteem etc.) needed to be constantly suffering and depressed as a way to placate or expiate the cruel and perverse superego. The narcissistic quality of this defence meant that Gloria felt compelled to surrender to the harsh superego rather than to challenge it or to accept anything good from an internal or external good object because this would interfere with her masochistic identification as the superego's victim.

By surrendering to the harsh superego Gloria deprived herself of the love and support of any internal and external good object and, combined with the criticisms coming from the harsh superego, she had no sources of love from which to revitalise her ego and find the necessary affection for the development of her self-esteem and prevent the onset of depression. To compensate for her inability to draw on the nourishment of any good objects she developed a narcissistic defence to protect her from the attacks of her superego. But at the same time this narcissistic defence deprived her of the necessary narcissistic real love her ego needed in order not to become depressed (Freud 1914). In healthy development, aggression helps the person to separate from their object and thus promotes psychic development

(Stewart 1992). In this case, Gloria could not use her aggression to help her to separate from her mother and foster her development, self-growth and self-love. Instead, she used her aggression to reject any object that would interfere with this defensive masochistic identification with her critical mother in an unsuccessful attempt to prevent the critical superego from attacking the ego for trying to separate from mother.

Intensive work on this highly critical internal world and its projections onto her analytic relationship with me partially transformed her harsh superego and freed some internal space in Gloria's mind (Stewart 1992). With this newly achieved inner freedom, we were able not only to help Gloria take good things from her objects, but also to recover some aspects of her private personal story and some material from her past life.

The main narrative in the historical reconstruction of her personal history and phantasies (Chianese 2004) were of a terrified little girl, who always felt unable to be herself or to be by herself. She remembered witnessing her mother's violent attacks on her younger sister, while she was desperately trying to be a good daughter and placate mother to avoid the attacks being directed at her. We also discovered within the descriptions of her personal narrative some powerful perverse phantasies and sadistic anal abusive wishes of her own, towards herself and others (Chianese 2004).

Gloria tried to cut herself off emotionally and psychologically from these violent experiences and phantasies of mother and herself, but when the mother's intrusive and abusive violent behaviour penetrated her psychological defences she fled South America. Gloria felt that she could only survive this powerful intrusive mother by escaping from her country and by developing an internal defence mechanism of cutting off. Unfortunately, although these defences saved Gloria from total collapse, they did not at the same time really work to foster a successful and creative internal and external life. At the time of starting her analysis Gloria was beginning to realise that 8000 miles' distance was not ameliorating her suicidal wishes or her disturbing murderous feelings or her infuriating conflictual relationship with her mother.

Gloria's critical self was a combination of her experience of a very intrusive ill mother and Gloria's own violent projections onto the internalisation of this mother. This critical part of her, like the mother, became an internal abuser, which, in turn, forced Gloria to split and develop a narcissistic personality structure to protect herself from this overpowering mother as a kind of self-preservative measure. In order to protect herself from the impingement and pain inflicted by her sadistic internal and external mother, my patient developed a narcissistic structure that unsuccessfully attempted to do two things at the same time: first, to protect her by allowing her to cut off from this violent intrusive critical mother, and, second, to nourish her by allowing her to unite in phantasy with the idealised mother she never had! Gloria's retreat to narcissism was a way to protect herself from being suffocated and annihilated by her traumatic and intrusive relationship with her sadistic internal and external mother. At the same time, her retreat to narcissism was a search for a good and idealised substitute mother to protect her, as her real mother had not, from frustration, anxiety and pain. But in building such a dangerous defensive structure, Gloria also isolated herself from the real world and from the real possibility of being looked after, taken care of and nourished by real people. It seems that, in Gloria's case, her narcissistic protection, originally necessary for her survival, ultimately became her illness! As Freud, in his paper 'On narcissism' said: 'A strong egoism is a protection against falling ill, but in the last resort we must begin to love in order not to fall ill, and we are bound to fall ill if in consequence of frustration we are unable to love!' (1914: 85).

When Gloria developed a narcissistic character structure to survive she also created a repetitive vicious circle, whereby she made the shadow of her sadistic mother fall on her (Freud 1917), leading her ultimately to emptiness, depression and psychic impoverishment. By not separating from her mother, Gloria retreated into a narcissistic union with an idealised version of a good mother and in doing that, in a paradoxical way, she also internalised a version of the cruel mother she so much wanted to run away from. This is shown in her dream of the twins being killed by a woman: part of her ego (one twin) aligned with the cruel internal mother (superego) did not really separate from the external mother either and consequently this part would attack and try to destroy the other part of her ego (the other twin) that identified with me and the work of analysis. When she did that, Gloria's already severely divided and depleted inner world became even more flat, empty and dead, a horrible place, from which Gloria felt suicide was the only way out.

Furthermore, by surrounding herself with a narcissistic skin Gloria made herself even less tolerant of pain, anxiety and frustration (Rosenfeld 1964). She thought she was protecting herself from her mother's impingements but in reality she made herself even more sensitive to frustration and anger and in this way also more prone to depression. In this sense, Gloria's depression was the result of a violent attack on the good object via herself, usually following a narcissistic injury inflicted on her by her analyst, whenever analytic work tried to dismantle this narcissistic configuration. For example, every time I interpreted, challenged her fusion with mother or confronted her cut-off-ness, Gloria experienced my intervention as a devastating narcissistic injury, with resulting loss of self-esteem and an internally violent emotional response. Her emotional violence confronted Gloria with an excruciating dilemma: she said, 'How can I hurt the only person who's helping me?' This intolerable dilemma plus the unbearable guilt she felt made Gloria direct in turn her violent feelings inward, mainly in the form of attacks on herself indirectly attacking me through attacking herself, via the internal identification of a part of herself with the analyst (Abraham 1924).

In order to protect her external mother and analyst from her narcissistic rage, Gloria would turn the attack into an inner battle with her internal mother and internal analyst, a battle that always left her feeling lonely, guilty, empty, depressed and suicidal.

Gloria's arrested ego development and incapacity for symbolisation

My starting point in this chapter was that Gloria's lack of imagination made her live in a constant state of violence and suffering. It is my contention that Gloria's passive-aggressive masochistic depression was connected with her lack of inner creative resources due to the severe and destructive critical part of Gloria's mind which impaired her symbolic function.

Zetzel has pointed out that 'the capacity to bear depression depends on the degree of development of the ego' (1965: 114). The capacity for happiness, learning and the development of object relations and the capacity to transform frustration and aggression into creative ego experiences without developing a narcissistic depression is contingent on the ego's ability to tackle its developmental tasks. Mastery of situations such as the inevitable frustrations and losses of life and of feelings, conflicts and relationships, depends on the ego's maturity and its capacity to master psychic functions and defences, in such a way that life's challenges can be faced in a flexible and creative way rather than in a regressive and destructive way. Psychic integration and maturity depends on the ego's capacity to integrate its experiences. Psychic integration is undermined by acute separation anxiety and explosive rage which impair the ego's capacity to integrate itself (Grinberg 1978). The creative personality is capable of tolerating frustration, chaos and disorder (Kleimberg 2003). However, when the ego is bombarded by overwhelming rage whenever it is confronted by frustration and loss and when the mother has not adequately contained the ego's early projections, the ego does not develop the capacity to integrate itself. Without integration the ego cannot properly separate from the object. Without the capacity to tolerate separation from the object the boundaries between self and object are lost and part of the object is confused with the ego. This undermines the ego's capacities to internalise, introject and identify with the object and impairs the development of the symbolic function (Segal 1991). The ego also depends on its capacity to introject and identify with the lost object as its primary ways to deal with loss; without these capacities the ego has very limited resources for coming to terms with loss of the object and frustration by the object (Freud 1917; Klein 1952).

The capacity for symbol formation is based on the ability to separate from the object, internalise its absence and form a mental representation of the object inside the mind in the absence of the object. When this happens the ego can relate to the object in its absence and become independent of the actual physical presence of the object. The capacity to relate to an object in its absence is the essence of the formation and functioning of the symbolic function. Transforming the absence into a presence in the mind is what gives the ego its symbolic function and its capacity to transform internal and external events and feelings into something 'else'. When this happens the something 'else' can be experienced in the internal and external world in a three-dimensional way. Segal (1991: 40–42) has described how, when the object is introjected by an ego that is severely split, the ego develops a more concrete version of this function, a symbolic equation, instead of developing a proper symbolic function. When the ego's capacity to symbolise is limited to the function of the symbolic equation as a result of restricted integration, the part-ego's identifications with the part-object is experienced in a concrete way: the symbol becomes the ego or the ego becomes the object. With a symbolic function parts of the self can be projected onto the introjected object without losing the comparative quality of the analogy (Grinberg 1978).With the symbolic equation the introjected object or parts of the object take over the notion of the self and give the self a sense of two-dimensionality and a sense of becoming like the introjected object in a concrete way (Grinberg 1978).

Gloria's ego development was severely restricted by the split and the narcissistic defensive system that was originally established to protect her and help her to survive a very disturbed intrusive mother. By creating a split inside herself between a good idealised mother (Rosenfeld 1964) and a cruel one and by investing, at the same time, a great deal of psychic energy in maintaining such a split, she could not allow any significant degree of integration in the self that could have facilitated the separation between her and the mother. It is important to note that, as is typical of these pathologies, the weak presence of the father and his unwillingness to intervene in this merger between Gloria and her mother contributed enormously to the impairment in Gloria's development of her symbolic function. Without a father to come between Gloria and her mother, or to turn to as an alternative to mother, Gloria was unable to develop the idea of a psychic space within her mind or the mind of others.

The separation that Gloria had not achieved is essential to foster the necessary healthy and contained processes of projective and introjective identifications, so important for the development of the symbolic function (Freud 1917; Grinberg 1978; Segal 1991) and consequently for the development of the capacity to play and imagine (Winnicott 1954; Zetzel 1965). Gloria could not develop emotionally and psychologically because of this. Her defence became her loss. Unable to move on from this vicious circle, she got stuck in a concrete, non-symbolic world where she could not develop the skills to deal with her aggression in a creative and imaginative way. She started *destroying* life rather than *giving* life. Her lack of imagination was not so much, I think, the kind of envious attack on the self that Rosenfeld

(1964) has described in his paper on the psychopathology of narcissism. Rather it was the result of Gloria's narcissistic attacks on her internal objects, through attacking herself (Abraham 1924) when her good objects challenged her defensive narcissistic skin and sado-masochistic merger with the mother.

Unable to separate from such a cruel mother, she was consequently unable to develop her ego sufficiently to perform the developmental tasks necessary for growth and maturity (Zetzel 1965). Gloria's underdeveloped and split ego did not have the strength to tolerate frustration, loss and guilt so that it could transform these experiences into a healthy depression, ultimately leading to an active adaptation to reality with creative solutions. Gloria's pathological depression resulted from a failure to transform her aggression and mobilise it to help her separate from mother. Gloria, unaided by father, and undermined by her mother, was not helped to make this developmental step. Without the capacity to separate from mother and represent her fully and symbolically in her mind Gloria was unable to become a person in her own right.

Instead, Gloria resorted to a symbolic equation, becoming the cruel mother herself and to herself in a kind of corrupted, psychotic concrete identification with mother. In her identification with her cruel internalised mother, she attacked her internal and external helpful objects preventing any intervention in the sado-masochistic fusion with the cruel internalised mother (Grinberg 1978). When she was not in identification with the sadistic internal and external mother and attacking her good objects, she herself became the object of attacks by this sadistic superego, which left her feeling excessively and overpoweringly guilty to the point of feeling extremely suicidal. By unconsciously choosing this way of trying to resolve her internal and external life demands, Gloria became trapped in a self-perpetuating destructive vicious circle.

By failing to separate from her mother Gloria remained stuck in a destructive depression resulting from her narcissistic attacks on the good and creative object. Quite clearly there was a price to pay for separating from mother, which was to incur mother's attacks, a price that Gloria was not prepared to pay. Her ego, unaided by father, was not integrated enough to go one step further on its own, and experience the loss of an object through separating from it and letting it have a life of its own (Grinberg 1978). Her depression was not the result of mournful feelings following the realisation of the loss or damage inflicted to the good internal creative object, ultimately the object that could have helped her to separate from her mother. When Gloria turned her attacks on the good aspects of mother and analyst inwardly, she undermined and destroyed even further what was valuable to her in her inner world. Her sense of emptiness resulted from her destructive attacks on the good and creative object within herself and her analyst.

This kind of pathological depression was like a vortex that would arrest her developmental progress and consistently undermine her ego growth (Kleimberg 2003). The creative process involved in psychic growth required Gloria to integrate the splits in her ego sufficiently to tolerate the frustration, anxiety and guilt that are inevitably evoked by learning and growing, and to survive the 'void' and state of 'disorder' and 'chaos' that a leap forward in development involves (Grinberg 1978). Gloria had not achieved this developmental step and consequently had not developed a symbolic function and stayed stuck at the level of a symbolic equation (Segal 1991) where she remained for many years unable to progress. Gloria was not able to do what Zetzel has so beautifully described of healthy children: 'Healthy children who do not fear life – in spite of subjective awareness of its limitations – will become adults with integrity enough not to fear death' (1965: 114).

Work on her incapacity to be creative and on her rigid sadistic superego freed Gloria from some of the restrictions that impaired her development. Some developmental achievement became possible once her ego was stronger and freer and capable of integrating itself and separating from her mother. The analyst and analysis acting as catalysts, or as the father (third object) Gloria did not have, also helped Gloria to break her entanglement with this engulfing mother, hence fostering further development and personal growth in her. This in turn allowed Gloria to recover some of the ego skills necessary to transform narcissistic reactive aggression into healthy separateness. This step enabled Gloria to undergo a more creative experience of depression and through this healthy depression she was able to acquire the appropriate and necessary ego resources to process and work through the different conflicts and feelings that she experienced as she separated from her mother and became aware of the loss and damage done to herself and others. These shifts inside Gloria's mind were indicated by a dream. In the dream, Gloria was with her mother in a corridor. Her mother was trying to attack Gloria but Gloria said to her mother: 'Do not try to attack me, you cannot hit me any more, you cannot hurt me any more.'

Gloria's ability to put boundaries between herself and her mother in the dream, as shown by the way she was able to stop her mother from abusing her, indicates that a psychic shift had taken place in Gloria's mind. Such a shift I believe is a reflection of the way she seems to have separated more from mother and caught up with further ego developments. Hopefully, this newly acquired maturity and integration will allow Gloria's imagination and creativity to continue transforming the 'black depression' or 'emptiness' from which she suffers and create more helpful ways to use her aggression. Perhaps Gloria is beginning to realise that using her aggression to separate from a sadistic mother is more creative than using her aggression to attack the helping and creative object inside herself.

Conclusion

A good example of the processes I have been describing in this chapter, albeit on a social dimension, is how the Mayor of Bogotá-Colombia dealt with the never ending cycle of violence, hatred and depression in the city. It seems that with his brave use of imagination in politics and civil administration he has managed to break a deadly vicious circle of violence and social depression in the city of Bogotá (*The Times*, London, September 2002). Apparently instead of meeting violence, murder and kidnapping with more reactive violence, as many politicians seem to do, he has introduced instead art exhibitions, decent libraries, women-only nights in the city twice a week and early closing hours for raucous restaurants. In an act of defiance and creativity, he seems to have stopped the spiralling violence, by also sending clowns and mime artists into the streets rather than an increased police force. He has become a symbol of civic resistance to violence and drug trafficking by refusing to use traditional violent means to deal with national endemic violence as other public authorities do. His courageous refusal to respond to violence with more narcissistic violence has allowed people in the city to recover their sense of creativity to process problems in a more inspired way, something that my patient Gloria was not able to do at the beginning of her analysis.

When Gloria started analysis, her ego was split into two parts. At the time one part of her ego became merged and fused in a corrupt and perverse way with the introject of a sadistic mother and the other part of her ego tried to adapt and placate this internal persecutory object in a submissive and servile way. With a split ego her symbolic function was reduced to the level of symbolic equation (Segal 1991). At this point her creativity and imagination were severely reduced and Gloria's capacity to symbolise, think, separate and find creative and mobile solutions to her restricted psychic and social life were severely impaired. Her restricted symbolic function rendered her unable to transform her hate and aggression into the emotional strength she needed in order to separate from this pathological identification; instead her hate and aggression remained unaltered and were used to attack Gloria's attempts to separate from mother. Whenever she tried to separate and have a life of her own, this destructive aggression made her feel criticised and guilty, truncating any attempt for further growth and development. This self-perpetuating concrete vicious circle, together with the restrictions on her internalisation of good and creative objects, deprived Gloria of the love she needed from the creative good object, consequently depleting her of the self-esteem she needed to withstand depression. The type of depression Gloria developed before her analysis was not of a mournful type, but a masochistic one. The masochistic depression she developed did not help Gloria to integrate herself and separate from mother. On the contrary, it was destructive, undermining and erosive, inhibiting her potential for development and creativity. She was trapped in a narcissistic defensive world, where her aggression was not used in the service of integration and health but rather used to protect the split she created to avoid the guilt and the sense of disintegration she would feel were she to separate from this pathological mother. Gloria's narcissistic and depressive world was a conundrum. If she did not separate from this pathological narcissistic identification, she would become masochistically depressed. If she were to try to separate from this narcissistic identification, she would become depressed and suicidal as a result of sadistic guilt and criticisms coming from her inappropriate and disturbed internal object.

The absence of separateness from the mother restricted the development of Gloria's symbolic function. The absence of symbolic function hindered her creative resources and the limitations in her creative processes prevented her from transforming aggression into healthy experiences.

The choice of such a pathological psychic solution is a paradox and a trap, in life as well as in clinical analysis. When patients choose this pathological dynamic, therapists and other professionals trying to help these patients are challenged by the question of how to break the sado-masochistic self-perpetuating vicious circle that this concrete pathological enclave represents, without becoming the abusive and sadistic internal and external object ourselves in the transference.

I hope that, as the Mayor of Bogotá was able to respond imaginatively to the violence in his city, so Gloria's emerging imagination will also eventually help her to replace hatred, violence and destruction with creativity, healthy anger, inspiration and growth, as Graham Greene (1940) suggested in *The Power and the Glory*.

References

Abraham, K. (1911) 'Notes on the psycho-analytical investigation and treatment of manic-depressive insanity and allied conditions' in *Selected Papers on Psychoanalysis*, London: Maresfield Library

—— (1924) 'A short study of the development of the libido, viewed in the light of mental disorders' in *Selected Papers on Psychoanalysis*, London: Maresfield Library

Chianese, D. (2004) *Construcciones y Campo Analitico, Buenos Aires*, Argentina: Grupo Editorial Lumen

Fenichel, O. (1946) 'Depression and mania' in *The Psychoanalytic Theory Of Neurosis*, London: Kegan Paul, Trench, Trubner & Co. Ltd

Freud, S. (1914) 'On narcissism: an introduction', *Standard Edition 14*, London: Hogarth Press

—— (1917) 'Mourning and melancholia', *Standard Edition 14*, London: Hogarth Press

—— (1926) 'The question of lay analysis', *Standard Edition 20*, London: Hogarth Press

Gay, P. (1995) *Freud: A Life for our Time*, London: Papermac

Greene, G. (1940) *The Power and the Glory*, Spain: Ed Plaza & Janes

Grinberg, L. (1978) 'The 'razor's edge' in depression and mourning', *International Journal of Psychoanalysis* 59: 245–54

Kleimberg, L. (2003) 'Cuidado con la ranura: psicoanalisis y creatividad . . . Y que pasa en el espacio en el medio!', *Revista Transiciones Appna* 6: 36–45

Klein, M. (1952) 'Some theoretical conclusions regarding the emotional life of the infant' in *Envy and Gratitude and Other Works*, London: Hogarth Press

Rosenfeld, H.A. (1964) 'On the psychopathology of narcissism: a clinical approach' in *Psychotic States*, London: Maresfield Reprints

Segal, H. (1991) *Dream, Phantasy and Art. The New Library of Psychoanalysis*, London: Routledge

Stewart, H. (1992) 'Changes in the experiencing of inner space' in *Psychic Experience and Problems of Technique*, E. Spillius (ed.), London: Karnac

Winnicott, D.W. (1954) 'The depressive position in normal emotional development' in *Through Paediatrics To Psycho-Analysis*, London: Hogarth Press

Zetzel, E.R. (1965) 'On the incapacity to bear depression' in *The Capacity for Emotional Growth*, London: Hogarth Press

Chapter 12

Destructive attacks on reality and the self

Richard Lucas

Introduction

In this chapter, I am going to focus on destructive attacks on reality and the self as experienced in the area of everyday general psychiatry. It will be shown how analytic insights can inform the underlying psychopathology and aid one's work in understanding and coping with tragedies related to violent acts towards self and others.

In working in general psychiatry, there are three areas of particular concern. There is violence directed at self (suicidal acts), violence directed at others (murderous attacks) and the effect of such incidents on staff morale. In contrast to other recent analytic contributions on violence (Perelberg 1999), I will be focusing here on the more extreme psychotic states of mind encountered in general psychiatry.

We need to develop frameworks of understanding to cope when we are presented with either potential or actual destructive actions. In working with patients with unpredictably fluctuating states of mind constant risk assessment is required (Lucas 2003). This chapter describes the author's development of frameworks of understanding linked to clinical experiences and how these contrast with a more prescriptive approach from management through the introduction of risk assessment forms.

The overall assessment of risk

In the last decade momentous changes have occurred within the National Health Service, with the closure of the large asylums and a shift of emphasis to community care in conjunction with district hospitals. Subsequent tragedies occurred, such as the Clunis case when a man with paranoid schizophrenia and a history of past aggression was left unsupervised in the community: in a deluded state he killed a stranger. Such tragedies led to the creation of more medium secure units but not more general psychiatric facilities.

Management's anxiety over containing disturbed behaviour has replaced asylum walls with 'walls of paper', namely the Care Programme Approach (CPA) form and the risk assessment form. The problem with forms can be that they encourage a psychotic belief that everything would have been all right if only one had followed the form. In contrast, review and research articles continue to reinforce the view that there is no foolproof way to prevent tragedies. Proulx, Lesage, and Grunberg (1997) in a study of 100 inpatient suicides concluded that: 'Inpatient suicides remain a relatively rare phenomenon difficult to predict, and that all the signs of a potentially impending suicide can be identified more easily with the benefit of hindsight.' If used retrospectively, suicide risk scales tended to identify a large number of false positives. Their study could not find any specific item that would improve the specificity of such scales.

However, the desire, emanating from government, to achieve an anxiety-free state in relation to potentially violent acts directed to self or others, has resulted in the irresistible momentum to give undue weight to risk assessment forms. The statistics from Appleby's National Confidential Inquiry into homicides and suicides revealed that 24 percent of suicide cases, some 1200, had previous contact with mental health services. Half of these had contact with mental health services in the week before death, but in 85 percent of cases the risk was not perceived. Among the recommendations for improvement was a thorough overhaul of the CPA and training in risk assessment (Appleby 1997; Thompson 1999). This preoccupation with forms seems a non-sequitur as the patients were actually receiving medical attention at the time of suicide. The proper conclusion is that when it comes to individual cases, we still have to rely on our own sensitivities and clinical acumen and learn from experience.

The following serves as an example of what I would call a delusional belief in the power of forms over feelings. It comes from a monthly trust review on violent incidents and the recommended lessons to be learned. It is typical of many others:

Incident: Doctor kicked on the shin while assessing a patient in the emergency reception centre.
Recommendation: Training on risk assessment required.
Lessons learnt: Completion of risk assessment forms on all patients.

Forms do have their uses. It is always important to record suicidal ideation in the medical or nursing notes. Perhaps the CPA's best feature is the requirement to designate a key worker responsible for coordinating follow-up care. The risk assessment's best feature is an invitation to look through past psychiatric records to alert one to previous alarming states of mind and acting-out behaviour. However, spending time filling out 120 boxes on a risk assessment form is not only unnecessary bureaucracy, but also takes valuable time away from the nurses' contact with their patients. Forms will never be a substitute for learning from actual clinical experience and acquiring relevant frameworks of understanding is an ongoing individual learning curve for all of us.

Destructive attacks on reality

In this section, I will outline my understanding of some of the analytic concepts that helped towards making sense of the presented clinical material.

In his seminal paper, 'On narcissism' (1914), Freud invited us to think about two quite distinctive and separate ways in which the mind works: the anaclitic and the narcissistic. The healthy anaclitic mind develops through introjecting parental figures and teachers on whom the person depends. In contrast, when narcissistic trends predominate in the mind, there is no psychic development, one takes one's self as love object and any needs for external objects are negated.

In major psychotic disorders, namely depression (melancholia) and schizophrenia, narcissistic trends predominate, leading Freud to regard psychoses as narcissistic neuroses. With his later introduction of an innate destructive drive (Freud 1920) one could now view narcissism as fuelled by the death instinct. In Kleinian terms, envy would be seen as the external manifestation of the death instinct. As Freud became aware of the power of narcissistic forces operating in psychoses, he became pessimistic about the prospect of forming a therapeutic relationship with psychotic patients and raised questions as to their capacity to respond to the analytic technique.

In 'Mourning and melancholia' (1917) Freud made further contributions to understanding the dynamics underlying psychotic depression. While mourning is linked to an external loss, the loss in depression is an unconscious, internal narcissistic loss. The patient wants to have his cake and eat it. He complains about losing an ideal, whenever a problem or illness arises, yet holds onto the concept that everything could still be perfect. When the depressed patient berates himself as no good, he is in identification with an ideal object that has let him down.

Freud describes the development of an extraordinarily harsh critical agency operating in depression later termed the superego (1923). He described how one part of the ego sets itself up against the other and judges it critically. Freud commented on the particular harsh nature of the superego operating in relation to melancholia, noting an 'extraordinary harshness and severity towards the ego' in both obsessional neurosis and melancholia. However, the superego is more dangerous in melancholia where it represents 'a pure culture of the death instinct . . . [which] often succeeds in driving the ego to death' (Freud 1923: 53).

In classical Freudian theory, the parental values are incorporated into the formation of the superego, with the resolution of the Oedipus Complex.

Klein described an early pre-oedipal stage to the formation of the superego, with a very harsh superego in evidence at the oral phase, which could become modified over time, with experience, to become more benign, less demanding and more tolerant towards human frailties (Segal 1973). However, Klein also referred to an early very harsh superego that stood apart and remained unmodified by the normal processes of growth, leading to consideration of a different superego operating in depression (Klein 1958; O'Shaughnessy 1999). Bion described the characteristics of this ego-destructive superego in the following way: 'It is a super-ego that has hardly any characteristics of the super-ego as understood in psychoanalysis: it is "super" ego. It is an envious assertion of moral superiority without any morals' (Bion 1962: 97). He further comments:

> In so far as its resemblance to the super-ego . . . shows itself as a superior object asserting its superiority by finding fault with everything. The most important characteristic is its hatred of any new development in the personality as if the new development were a rival to be destroyed.
>
> (1962: 98)

Bion's hypothesis was that the pathological superego arose out of early failures in communication between the infant and mother. In depression, the ego-destructive superego will occupy the driving seat and attack the self. In such a situation, O'Shaughnessy summarises:

> No working through can take place, only an impoverishment and deterioration of relations, with an escalation of hatred and anxiety that results in psychotic panic or despair. In this dangerous situation, the significant event for the patient is to be enabled to move away from his abnormal superego, return to his object, and so experience the analyst as an object with a normal superego.
>
> (1999: 861)

Freud also described our first ego as a bodily ego. In other words, our first sensations are bodily ones and we bring in the mind to cope with physical deprivation, e.g. sucking one's thumb to hallucinate a comforting breast. Therefore, from birth, an intimate relationship exists between the body and the mind. At different times we project the good object or the bad object, or a mixture of the two, into the body, reflecting our varying attitudes to our body.

Klein described how the infant initially splits their object into the good and bad object, idealising the good object to protect it from projected envious attacks. In healthy development, in the more reflective states of the depressive position, the good and bad objects come together and become seen as part of a more whole object. If persecutory guilt about damaging the good object is too much to bear then regression into paranoid-schizoid states can occur (Segal 1973). The bad object may then become installed in the body and be the subject of attack to preserve the good object, as in some adolescents who cut themselves to experience relief from tension (Laufer & Laufer 1984).

However, when considering destructive attacks in major psychotic disorders, depression and schizophrenia, it is the destructive, narcissistically driven, psychotic part, not the good object, that is to be preserved from attack. When the psychotic part feels threatened, it turns on the sane part that has been projected into the body. Bell summarises this dynamic in a paper addressing the internal phenomenology of the suicide act: 'The body that has been attacked in a suicidal act is a body that has become identified with a psychic object that cannot be tolerated' (Bell 2001: 21).

To understand this dynamic further, we may turn to Bion's contributions to our understanding of psychotic disorders. He describes two parts to the personality, the psychotic and non-psychotic. These are quite separate in their functioning, to my mind extending Freud's view of the narcissistic and anaclitic parts (Bion 1957). The psychotic part, fuelled by the death instinct, from early in life, attacks the perceptual apparatus, i.e. the part of the mind that is needed to register and evaluate feelings. The psychotic part of the mind lacks the capacity to learn from experience. Instead, it acts like a muscular organ evacuating the feelings arrived at through the work of the non-psychotic part. The psychotic part wants everything to be trouble free and tries to achieve this by creating an omnipotent delusion of perfection. It is in endless rivalry with the non-psychotic part, which is under the sway of the life instinct and is linked with learning from experience.

Bion (1957) invites us to assess whether a communication is a straightforward communication from the non-psychotic part or a rationalisation from the psychotic part. I recall Bion once saying that he was at an advantage when he heard Hitler on the radio before the war because, not understanding German, he was not seduced by Hitler's rationalisations and could recognise the psychotic nature of Hitler's mental state from the tone of his voice. The psychotic part only has mathematical logic at its disposal to address problems pertaining to the emotional sphere. A striking illustration of this was a patient with chronic schizophrenia, who decided that he wanted to leave hospital and have sex, so he applied to the YWCA for a vacancy. He signed his letter 'the World's Best Logician'. When told that the hostel was not mixed sex and asked to consider his actions, he saw no problem, because the hostel would be a mixed one if he lived in it. His logic was impeccable, but it missed out all the related emotional aspects. The commonest symptoms of psychosis are, in fact, not hallucinations and delusions, occurring in 60 percent of cases, but denial and rationalisation occurring in over 95 percent, which may lead to a serious underestimation of the severity of the underlying psychosis (Gelder, Gath, Mayou, & Cowen 1998).

To summarise, when relating to destructive attacks on reality associated with major psychiatric disorders, one needs to think in terms of two separate parts to the personality and to bear in mind that the psychotic part is the dominating force. It is resistant to change and, at times of feeling under threat, can produce a dangerous backlash. Since there is an intimate relationship between the mind and the body, the non-psychotic sane part can be projected into the body and the body then attacked. This situation, arising in major psychotic disorders, is to be distinguished from borderline states, where a suffocating object might be projected into the body and temporary relief of tension sought through cutting.

Violence to self

The selected analytic concepts just outlined helped promote understanding of suicidal states of mind aiding us in our efforts to keep our anxieties, and those of staff, relatives and management, within manageable proportions. The following two examples illustrate how experience gained from one suicide helped to make sense of a subsequent suicide through the application of this framework for understanding.

An inpatient suicide

Mrs X was a middle-aged woman with a 10-year history of unremitting chronic severe psychotic depression. Many years ago, she had jumped on a railway line and lost both legs. Since then, she had made further suicide attempts by taking overdoses. Following the overdoses, she was admitted into hospital on section. She would never discuss her suicide attempts. She would just fixate me with a chillingly murderous stare. She would also have screaming fits on the ward that were not amenable to discussion, but would subside prior to discharge back into the community.

We spoke at length with her husband about her outlook and how one day she was likely to kill herself. We agreed we could only do our best. While in hospital, the nursing staff and occupational therapist found it hard to engage her in any activity. The only sign of life she gave was her interest in playing games of Scrabble. Linked with my counter-transference feelings of being at the receiving end of the chilling stare, I understood the underlying dynamics in terms of a dominating murderous psychotic part keeping imprisoned another part of her wanting human contact, i.e. through the games of Scrabble.

In other words, as already described, it is important here to think about two totally separate parts to the personality. There is a powerful psychotic part. Its features are that it is never to be contradicted. Fuelled by the death instinct, nothing is allowed to change or develop. It is never to be challenged or criticised, and any attempt to change this state of affairs will lead to a murderous backlash. It keeps imprisoned another part of the personality, the non-psychotic part that wants companionship and support for development and freedom of expression. My counter-transference experience at the time alerted me to the underlying dynamic of a powerful psychotic part keeping the non-psychotic part in an imprisoned state.

When she returned home, Mrs X tended to lie downstairs with her elderly mother in attendance until the next admission. I put to her that there was an imprisoned part of her mind that wanted us to help bring some variety into her life when out of hospital and a tear trickled down her cheek. She said that she would like to be taken swimming. We said that we would make arrangements for a befriender to take her swimming when she was settled enough to return home. The CPA programme was fully in place and recorded.

Two weeks before her death, she was left behind while other patients went on a day trip by bus to the seaside because the bus could not accommodate her wheelchair. She appeared angry. Afterwards, when having a bath, the nurse bathing her left her briefly to fetch a towel. The nurse returned to find her submerged under water giving the nurse a fright as she pulled her up. This bathroom also contained the only toilet on the ward wide enough to accommodate her wheelchair from which she could get independently onto the toilet. Her mood settled over the next 24 hours. She continued, as previously, to go independently to that toilet. Within two weeks, it was felt that she was ready for a trial weekend at home. Her husband came on the Saturday morning to collect her. She had gone to the toilet. While there she turned on the bath and drowned herself.

The reactions to this event are of particular interest. I had been away on leave and returned to face an internal hospital inquiry to investigate and look for any lessons to be learned. For example, was the CPA form completed and had it been reviewed recently? Did everyone know its content? Did another nurse become the key worker if the key worker was not on duty? Was there adequate interdisciplinary communication? Could the ward be altered in design to enhance safety? However, with the anxiety engendered and pressures to produce a report with recommendations, there is a danger that these sorts of question become regarded as possible explanations for the tragedy. The nursing staff who had cared for the patient and were devastated by her death, gave flowers and went to her funeral, inevitably then experienced themselves as if on the receiving end of a clinical inquiry.

Freud described in all of us both self-preservative life forces and self-destructive forces, the latter being linked with his concept of an innate death instinct (Freud 1920). Usually our emotional states contain a mixture of positive and negative feelings. However, at times of suicidal and violent acts, there is a diffusion of the two forces, with the destructive force in the ascendancy. It may also be helpful to think in Bion's terms of two separate parts the psychotic and non-psychotic part (Bion 1957). In some cases of suicide, one might view the psychotic part of the mind as killing the non-psychotic part, to avoid having to account for its own destructiveness. One might look at the inpatient suicide I described in those terms, i.e. the more open, healthy state of mind emerging with her tears making her vulnerable to a deadly defensive backlash.

In his classical paper 'Mourning and melancholia', Freud described how we all have to go through the work of mourning after the loss of loved ones (Freud 1917). We have to accept their death and through mourning we reinstate them inside us in our memory. The finality of the suicide act, however, inclines us more to melancholic reactions, attributing blame to ourselves or others due to the unbearable pain of the situation. The super-ego plays a leading role at every stage of the process from the patient's illness and suicide to the consequences afterwards and for the participants at every level of involvement, the family, the consultant and other profes-sionals and the organisations involved.

As the consultant, I saw my role as offering support to the nursing staff by attempting to bring in a balanced perspective; namely, that while an inquiry must be made and any lessons learned, the tragedy was nobody's fault and could not have been prevented. It was interesting to consider my superego or critical conscience, which I felt answerable to in that situation, as the consultant. In my mind, the arbitrator would be an understanding coroner.

Unfortunately, as illustrated in this and the next case, it is not always possible to enable the patient to reinstate the more benign superego, and prevent the deathly attack on the ego. In this case, the coroner represented the reinstatement of a more benign mature reflective superego that tolerated the complexities of life, rather than blaming the staff.

All suicides challenge our omnipotent beliefs that we can help everyone and could have prevented tragedies if only we had carried out the right practice, exposing those involved to the accusations from harsh superego representations. Suicides are particularly hard on nursing staff, who gave loving care to a patient over many admissions, to try to come to terms with a suicide, while having to answer an immediate internal inquiry centred on CPA and risk assessment forms. Fortunately, in this case, the coroner proved to be non-judgemental. He, in fact, apportioned no blame or criticism, just sympathy to all those affected by the tragedy. Coming up to me afterwards, he gave the opinion that he felt that her condition was untreatable.

A suicide in the community

The preceding experience helped me when having to face an even more horrendous situation. Mr Y was a man of 39 years. His psychiatric notes described two brief admissions in his early 20s in a paranoid state. He was given a diagnosis of schizophrenia and placed on depot medication, which he had taken ever since. He had never worked. His father died many years ago and for decades he lived with his mother. Recently there was a suggestion of mild mood swings. There had been no admissions for over 15 years. He had no history of self-harm.

Mr Y had a very supportive family of four sisters and a brother and a community mental health nurse (CMHN) monitoring the situation. He preferred to do his own thing rather than attend a day centre. When his mother died he moved into joint accommodation with his single brother, who went to work. He would visit his sisters during the day and one married sister was particularly supportive.

He moved into our catchment area and it was noted that he had developed an agitated depression. His CMHN became concerned and felt that he needed medical attention and she referred him to me. I saw him in the middle of a busy new patient clinic. He was clearly in an agitated preoccupied state. However, while accepting antidepressant medication, he refused an offer of admission. He also refused the offer of attending the day hospital, saying that he would think about it. He denied any suicidal feelings, but conveyed a distressed state and he was also informed of the emergency reception centre facility.

I did not think at the time that he was sectionable or that his family would have supported admission. I therefore arranged to review him at my next outpatient clinic, and told him to bring along a relative. Although he was clearly unwell, he refused all offers of help before I had to terminate the interview.

On Monday morning I was informed of his suicide on the previous Friday afternoon. He came to the hospital on Friday midday to collect his tablets and bumped into his CMHN, who used the opportunity to check on his mental state. He had not slept the night before, but then had slept to midday. When asked he denied feeling suicidal. She advised him to go round to his sister, until his brother returned from work. His brother had also ascertained that Mr Y had not slept the night before, advised him to sleep to midday and then go round to his sister. Again he denied suicidal feelings. When he returned from work that afternoon, his brother found Mr Y lying dead, with blood everywhere. He had cut his throat, wrists, body and legs and had walked round the flat until he died. There was an open empty medicine bottle on the floor.

Mr Y's suicide was a severe shock to both professionals and relatives. His eldest sister rang up saying that the family wanted help to understand and make sense of it. They did not blame anyone. I was left trying to process this on a typical very demanding NHS Monday morning. In the midst of my many commitments, as the consultant, I had to cope with my own feelings of guilt, with the immediate effect on the supporting staff and attempt to process and make sense of the tragedy for the meeting arranged with Mr Y's family and CHMN.

I had to come to an understanding of what had happened that would convince me and help Mr Y's relatives. In my formulation, I drew on my experience from the inpatient suicide and the love from the nurses who attended the funeral and sent flowers. My understanding was based on the idea that the suicidal patient splits mind and body, equates the healthy part of the mind with the bad object and projects it into their body. Their body becomes identified with the bad object, which is then murderously attacked (Bell 2001). I brought in the split between two parts of the patient's mind, the healthy part, which responded to his family's love and appreciated their love and care, and the ill, very secretive part that had hidden his suicidal intentions.

The suicide of a relative is beyond ordinary comprehension and empathy alone was not enough. I had to help the relatives to understand that the patient, on reaching mid-life, separated from his mother, was having to face up to the destructiveness of the psychotic part of his mind and how it had prevented him from living. When internally brought to account, the psychotic part murderously attacked the evidence by killing itself. It was interesting on sharing these thoughts with his sisters that one recalled the patient saying three months previously: 'My body is tired of living.' I was then able to share with them my own counter-transference feelings of guilt and helplessness. These understandings enabled the relatives to begin to express more ordinary guilt feelings, i.e. 'If only I'd done that' and to understand how he had been sick and why he appeared to have rejected all their love and support.

On this occasion, unlike the previous clinical example of Mrs X, the family and I had not been sufficiently aware of the patient's underlying murderous state of mind prior to the tragedy. After seeing the patient in outpatients, I was only left with a feeling of general unease and impatience over his having presented in a distressed state, while resistant to accepting offers of help. Only after the suicide was I able to recognise how destructive he had been and the compulsion to destroy that recognition. I then found myself able to draw on the experience with the previous patient, with the two separate parts of the personality, to help make sense of what had happened. The non-psychotic part had wanted to seek help and protection from the psychotic part, with its destructive force. The balance between the two forces led to the counter-transference feeling of an impasse towards making any progress, when trying to clarify his presenting state of mind. This time I did not have such a clear picture of an imprisoned part, as through projection I also felt imprisoned in the impasse.

Only after the tragedy, with wisdom of hindsight, was I able to fully appreciate the experience that I had undergone.

I was left feeling gratitude to analytic thinking, which, together with my previous experience, had helped me to arrive at a formulation that proved helpful to the relatives. I was, of course, still left with my own superego telling me that if you had spent more time with your patient or had been more sympathetic it may not have happened.

It is not surprising to hear about burnout and early retirement from general psychiatric posts or psychiatrists opting for quieter specialities with less demanding workloads. However, analytic thinking offers invaluable support and understanding, while continuing to work in the 'impossible profession'.

Violence to others – identifying the psychotic wavelength

Many interesting statistics have arisen from the National Confidential Inquiry into homicides and suicides in people with mental illness (Appleby 1997; Thompson 1999). Of the homicides, the majority had personality disorders, often abetted by drug or alcohol abuse, fewer had schizophrenia. Most victims were from within the family or someone they knew. However, within the field of general psychiatry, it is the patients with psychosis that present the challenge, when trying to determine the risk of potential violence. The violent act might be to a complete stranger. If persecutory or depressive feelings become unbearable, in the psychotic state, the patient may project the problem concretely into a stranger and then seek relief through attacking the stranger. Sohn described the process in detail with an analytic study of patients who attempted to push strangers onto railway lines (Sohn 1997).

While risk assessment takes place every time a patient with a history of psychosis is seen clinically, there are two particular settings where this is the central feature of the proceedings. These are when assessing the grounds for a formal hospital admission and when a hospital tribunal is considering whether it is safe to lift the restriction order.

The admission of a patient on a compulsory basis under the Mental Health Act requires a recommendation from two doctors. Ideally, one should be the patient's general practitioner (GP) who knows the patient well, and the other should be a specialist in psychiatry, ideally the responsible consultant. The approved social worker (ASW), after speaking with the nearest relative and seeing the patient, then decides whether to complete the section. In most cases, full agreement must be reached on the necessity for a formal admission. Only in cases where problems have arisen can lessons be learned. The following case serves as an illustration.

Case example 1

The mother of a patient with a previous record of admission in a violent psychotic state noted that her son seemed to be deteriorating. He had stopped complying with his medication. He would no longer allow her access to his residence and she noted, through his window, broken dishes in his bedroom. His mother notified the community mental health nurse (CMHN). The patient threatened to harm the CMHN if she attempted to visit.

The CMHN notified the GP and, as the responsible psychiatric consultant, I was requested to make a domiciliary visit. The patient was clearly in a guarded and paranoid state, only allowing a limited dialogue in the hallway. I completed my part of a compulsory order. The GP did not visit, as the patient's current residence was some distance from his practice. The ASW came with another doctor, approved under the act but unfamiliar with the patient previous to the visit. The patient was still guarded in manner, refusing access to his room arguing that one's privacy should be respected. He described his mother as having a poor understanding of his needs, but agreed that he should not have spoken threateningly to the CMHN.

The patient assured the ASW that he would visit his GP that week to collect further medication and would comply with outpatient attendance. In such a situation, it was felt that the order could not be completed. The ASW also suggested that the mother might benefit from some help to improve her understanding of her son. The next day he was formally admitted following an unprovoked violent attack towards a stranger in the community. He had thrown bleach in the face of a young woman waiting to collect her child from a school opposite to where he lived, fortunately, causing no permanent disfiguration or blindness. His stated wish at the time had been to scar her. A way of understanding his action was that the psychotic part wished to be free from involvement in self-reflection on his current mental state. He envied the child who seemingly had no problems as he was going to be totally looked after by his mother. The psychotic part wished to ensure that any current self-criticism of its state of mind was disowned and projected into the mother and attacked in her so that the psychotic part could remain in an omnipotent state of mind.

This brief vignette raises several issues for consideration aside from the immediate points that the GP who knew the patient was not able to be part of the assessment team and that the ASW had not spoken directly with the consultant before arriving at his decision.

Patients with psychotic disorders project and disown their problematic states of mind, especially when relapsing. As already noted, the most common presenting symptom of psychosis is not hallucinations or delusions but lack of insight presenting as denial and rationalisation (Gelder, Gath, Mayou & Cowen 1998). Bion's theory provides an analytic framework to help our understanding of this vignette. While the non-psychotic part of the mind is capable of reflection, the psychotic part, fuelled by envy and hatred of psychic reality, operates by evacuating troublesome feelings, thereby creating hallucinations and delusions. The psychotic part then covers up its murderous activity, through appearing calm and reasonable. Each time we have to make an assessment on a patient with a suggested history of psychosis, we consider whether we are hearing a straightforward communication from the non-psychotic part or a rationalisation from the psychotic part.

In physical illnesses, it is the doctor who makes the diagnosis. With relapse of psychosis, it is the relative who makes the diagnosis. Then it is a case of whether the professionals believe the relatives or the patient's denial of illness and rationalised explanations for his reported disturbed behaviour. Without Bion's model in mind, one may be forced into a position, as occurred in this case, of adopting a moral stance where the relative is held to be in the wrong and consequently the degree of the patient's potential violence is underestimated.

The other place where risk assessment in relation to potential violence arises is at mental health tribunals where a patient appeals against continuing detention in hospital. Tribunals can get into dreadful muddles if they do not recognise a separate psychotic part of the patient's mind, which is capable of disguise and rationalisation.

Case example 2

The parents of a patient eventually had him admitted to hospital because he was living as a recluse at home, refusing to collect his benefits and his parents had to do everything for him. His room was in such a state of neglect that they had to remove the door and replace it with a curtain to gain access to clean it. He had the delusion that he was a film producer. He would say that he had a team under him but would never be able to substantiate it. In hospital, he dressed soberly, with sports jacket and tie and his assertions sounded convincing. When he appealed against his section he insisted that his parents did not attend the tribunal. The tribunal sat for five hours but could not make up their minds about whether or not he was a film producer as he claimed. They adjourned pending the patient bringing in a film and asking for a professional film producer to come and evaluate it.

I attended a second outside tribunal. His parents were heard and the section was upheld. The case illustrates again the powerful persuasiveness of rationalisation and that the relatives' views must be obtained and carefully considered in all cases of risk assessment relating to psychosis. The very powerful projective identification of the madness into the listener results in the listener feeling that *they* must be mad because the other person seems so rational. One is then left either having to negate one's doubts or seek help from others who know more about the person's background and history.

Conclusion

Forms alone are not the way forward in risk assessment. Each presenting clinical case requires assessment in their own right and we have to rely on our own sensitivities and clinical acumen and learn what we can from unforeseen tragedies, as evidenced by the clinical illustrations. A review of major inquiries concluded that most tragedies were 'inherently unpredictable' (Blom-Cooper 1995). Good practice relied on good morale, in other words, the management and clinicians needed to support and respect each other and work as a team. A good working relationship between the involved members of the clinical team is the most important factor when trying to reduce the risk of tragedies, although it is not always possible to prevent them from happening. When tragedies occur, the team of professionals need to make sense of the situation and support each other and the relatives.

The aim of this chapter has been to demonstrate how analytic insights on the working of the mind have an important contribution to make in the individual assessment of dangerous states of mind. This way of thinking can then be shared with the team to aid in their deliberations. Continued development of our own analytic sensitivities and clinical skills remain the real challenge in the field of risk assessment.

References

Appleby, L. (1997) 'Progress report, National Confidential Inquiry into suicide and homicide by people with a mental illness', London: Department of Health

Bell, D. (2001) 'Who is killing what or whom? Some notes on the internal phenomenology of suicide', *Psychoanalytic Psychotherapy* 15: 21–37

Bion, W.R. (1957) 'Differentiation of the psychotic from non-psychotic personalities' in *Second Thoughts, Selected Papers on Psycho-analysis*, New York: Jason Aronson

—— (1962) '-K. Learning from experience' in *Seven Servants*, New York: Jason Aronson

Blom-Cooper, L. (1995) *The Falling Shadow: One Patient's Mental Health Care. 1978–1993*, London: Duckworth

Freud, S. (1914) 'On narcissism: an introduction', *Standard Edition 14*, London: Hogarth Press

—— (1917) 'Mourning and melancholia', *Standard Edition 14*, London: Hogarth Press

—— (1920) 'Beyond the pleasure principle', *Standard Edition 18*, London: Hogarth Press

—— (1923) 'The ego and the id', *Standard Edition 19*, London: Hogarth Press

Gelder, M., Gath, D., Mayou, R. and Cowen, P. (1998) *Oxford Textbook of Psychiatry*, 3rd edn, Oxford: Oxford University Press

Klein, M. (1958) 'On the development of mental functioning' in *Writings of Melanie Klein*, Vol. 3, London: Hogarth Press

Laplanche, J. and Pontalis, J.B. (1973) *The Language of Psycho-Analysis*, London: Hogarth Press

Laufer, M. and Laufer, M.E. (1984) 'Attempted suicide in adolescence: a psychotic episode', *Adolescence and Developmental Breakdown*, London: Karnac

Lucas, R. (2003) 'Risk assessment in general psychiatry: a psychoanalytic perspective', *Dangerous Patients. A Psychodynamic Approach to Risk Assessment and Management*, R. Doctor (ed.), London: Karnac

Morgan, G., Buckley, C. and Nowers, M. (1998) 'Face to face with the suicidal', *Advances in Psychiatric Treatment* 4: 188–96

O'Shaughnessy, E. (1999) 'Relating to the superego', *International Journal of Psychoanalysis* 80: 861–70

Perelberg, J.R. (1999) *Psychoanalytic Understanding of Violence and Suicide*, The New Library Series of Psychoanalysis, London: Routledge

Proulx, F., Lesage, A.D. and Grunberg, F. (1997) 'One hundred in-patient suicides', *British Journal of Psychiatry* 171: 247–50

Segal, H. (1973) *Introduction to the Work of Melanie Klein*, London: Hogarth Press

Sohn, L. (1997) 'Unprovoked assaults. Making sense of apparently random violence' in *Reason and Passion. A Celebration of the Work of Hanna Segal*, D. Bell (ed.), Tavistock Clinic Series, London: Duckworth

Stengel, E. (1946) *Suicide and Attempted Suicide*, London: Penguin

Thompson, C. (1999) 'The confidential inquiry comes of age', *British Journal of Psychiatry* 175: 301–2

Chapter 13

'Poison his delight': destructiveness and the ending of treatment

Anne Amos

In his play *Othello*, Shakespeare brings to life the feelings of envy, jealousy, love and hate and shows how they manifest themselves in intimate relationships. Iago knowingly and cruelly destroys Othello's love for his new wife Desdemona. Othello's love is turned into possessive and controlling jealousy. In the end, Othello kills Desdemona in order to possess her and in his guilt and regret he kills himself as well. Othello is driven by jealousy, a wish to hold onto a loved object, whereas Iago's motives are altogether different. He is possessed by envy, a wish to damage and spoil that which he himself can not possess. His intentions are made clear in his first speech of the play. When he hears of Othello and Desdemona's coupling, Iago encourages his henchman to stir up and incite Desdemona's father, who is protective of his daughter and inclined to be prejudiced against Othello as a 'Moor', saying,

> Call up her father,
> Rouse him: make after him, poison his delight,
> Proclaim him in the streets; incense her kinsman,
> And though he in a fertile climate dwell,
> Plague him with flies: though that his joy be joy,
> Yet throw such chances of vexation on't
> As it may lose some colour.
>
> (*Othello*, Act 1, Scene 1)

Iago is out to spoil. He is concerned that if Desdemona's father is to have any pleasure at his daughter's unusual, potentially interesting and fertile marriage it is to be poisoned and plagued with flies.

What provokes Iago, one of Shakespeare's most unpleasant characters, and makes him so unremittingly vicious at a deeper level is unclear. Within the play, the only explanation is that he feels slighted and downgraded by Othello when he is given a domestic and supporting role rather than a commanding position in Othello's army. He takes this as a slight on his person, which provokes the most terrible revenge that inflates throughout the play to the point where it can only be satisfied by the annihilation of Othello and Desdemona. Iago never seems to doubt his course of action for a moment. In fact, he revels in it, enjoying the secrecy and the power. Strikingly, the excitement he feels neither interferes with nor hinders his cold-blooded plan to destroy Othello. By contrast, Othello's fragile sense of himself and lack of confidence in Desdemona as a good figure leaves him naive and vulnerable and he is too easily tricked by Iago into doubting Desdemona's love for him. His love for her is poisoned and turns to hatred following her supposed rejection and humiliation of him.

I suggest that in our patients there is an Iago-like aspect of themselves that may hijack doubt. Similar to the way in which Othello doubts whether Desdemona loves him and he becomes confused and jealous, our patients too can become confused about whether their analyst is a good or a bad figure and whether the analytic method itself can be trusted. To depend on the person of the psychoanalyst or psychotherapist and the psychoanalytic method is to be in a very vulnerable position. I suggest it is this vulnerability, Othello-like, together with envy, Iago-like, that can combine together to make a deadly attack on the treatment itself and therefore the potential for development of the patient within the treatment. In some ways, the very nature of the psychotherapeutic or psychoanalytic task and process that has no obvious tangible or material gain makes it a particularly easy target for this sort of attack. It is expecting a great deal to sustain a psychotherapist or psychoanalyst as a good figure in the patient's mind when they are seen for 50 minutes between once and five times a week. The intense and elusive emotional contact in psychotherapy is therefore fertile ground for an Iago-like pernicious attack. The Iago-like aspects of our patients, when driven by envy or hatred of what the psychoanalyst has, can become big and cruel, torturing and tormenting, growing on its own success and only provoked further by encountering more need, vulnerability or doubt. Furthermore this aspect of the patient can be kept hidden and secret, in just the way that Othello was so unaware of Iago's dark side, believing him to be a good and trusted friend. This secrecy can be a way of feeling big and powerful to defend against the experience of actually feeling dependent on the psychoanalyst and the psychoanalytic method.

Psychoanalysts have long been concerned with the conflict between love and hate (life instincts and death instinct). While there continues to be controversy regarding the existence of a primordial death instinct what is clear, from the clinical field, is the way in which any achievement in treatment can potentially be unravelled through the process of what Freud (1923) termed the negative therapeutic reaction. In 'Analysis terminable and interminable' (1937), Freud directly linked the negative therapeutic reaction with the death instinct, suggesting that in some patients the ego has characteristics that resist treatment and that these 'spring from different and deeper roots'. He proposes that while this force, the death instinct, which resists treatment, has only a portion of it bound, or kept in check, by the superego, 'other quotas of the same force . . . may be at work in other *unspecified places*' (1937: 242–3, emphasis added). Freud is pointing to an aspect of our inner worlds that reacts to development and seem to the therapist to come from another place in the patient's mind.

With the understanding developed from the work of Klein by her followers, in particular Bion (1967), Rosenfeld (1986) and Segal (1993) in their treatment of psychotic patients, the malignant processes taking place in the mind have been further elucidated.

Segal (1993) begins her seminal paper 'On the clinical usefulness of the concept of the death instinct' with a quote from Jack London's *Martin Eden*: when Martin attempts suicide by drowning, he experiences an automatic wish to swim as he sinks which he treats with a sneer of disdain: '"The hurt was not death" was the thought that oscillated through his [Martin's] reeling consciousness. It was life – the pangs of life – this awful suffocating feeling. It was the last blow life could deal him.' Segal writes that 'all pain comes from living' and suggests that birth confronts us with an experience of need to which there are two basic reactions: one is to seek to satisfy the need (life instinct), while the other is to annihilate both the perception of needing and the object who could satisfy that needing feeling (death instinct). She suggests that in healthy development the conflicts of the life and death instincts are mainly under the aegis of the life instinct. In contrast, when the death instinct is predominant any appetite for life or development is hampered. For example, when Martin Eden is committing suicide, he has to resist the automatic wish to swim and he does this by treating that wish to swim with contempt therefore he stops himself from swimming and thereby from saving his own life. Segal suggests that in each of us, there is a delicate balance between these life and death forces and that the particular pattern of defences against the death instinct can lead to much psychopathology.

The process of psychoanalytic treatment itself unsettles the patient's psychic equilibrium, the delicate balance of life and death forces. Treatment is an attempt to free the patient from the constraints of their own minds and to enable them to engage in life more fully, it is about life and development and may provoke the more destructive sides of the personality, as exemplified by Martin Eden's 'sneer'. The features of destructive processes that become manifest in a psychoanalytic treatment are often understood to have been harnessed in 'pathological organisations' of the personality (O'Shaughnessy 1981; Steiner 1993). The pathological organisation of the mind is a structured pattern of impulses, anxieties and defences that traps the personality neither fully in the chaos of a psychotic world nor engaging in the emotional cost and difficulty of real emotional and psychic development. There is a debate as to whether the formation of an organisation that structures this destructiveness is of itself destructive or whether it is a defence against psychosis. I would suggest, following Spillius (1988), that it is both. Spillius (1988: 196) points out that it is implicit in the writings of authors such as Rosenfeld, Bion and Segal that 'these organisations are compromise formations, that is, that they are simultaneously expressions of death instinct and defences against it'.

Rosenfeld (1986), for example, describes a destructive process, similar to Segal (1993) that operates in the mind and becomes manifest in treatment. He calls this process 'destructive narcissism' and suggests that it often leads to a therapeutic impasse or stalemate between the patient and analyst. Destructive narcissism, he suggests, is the idealisation of the omnipotent, destructive parts of the self that come to dominate certain patients and cause them to want to destroy the analyst who stands for an object who has something good to offer the patient, a way of freeing themselves from their own mental constraints and therefore to enable emotional growth and development. Rosenfeld shows that in patients for whom destructive narcissism prevails, the whole self becomes identified with a destructive part that aims to triumph over life and creativity, like Martin Eden's sneer at his wish to swim and prevent himself from drowning (Segal 1993) and Iago's hatred of Othello and Desdemona's coupling. When these patients begin to feel that their analyst has something to offer them, they become aware of feelings of dependency and need along with the progress in their analysis. A severe negative therapeutic reaction to these new developments may occur when the narcissistic psychotic, destructive part of the self is provoked to exert its power anew and to lure the part of the self that is developing in the therapeutic endeavour and feeling more dependent and vulnerable into a psychotic, omnipotent dreamlike state where there is no pain of living. In this state, the patient can lose their sense of reality and capacity for thinking, creating, in effect, a kind of psychotic breakdown. Rosenfeld sees these patients as attempting to deal with their conflict between life and death instincts, which are re-opened in treatment, by totally identifying with their destructive propensities. It is as if their Iago-like propensities are unleashed in the face of the fragility of their development, just as Othello's fragile sense of self and ability to love did not sustain him in the face of Iago's poisoning. Destructive narcissism is for Rosenfeld a form of undiffused death instinct that provides the personality with a sense of superiority and self-admiration at the expense of real life and real development.

My clinical illustrations show the way these destructive processes, fuelled by the death instinct and structured in pathological organisations of the mind, attacked and destroyed the analytic treatment. I will illustrate with three clinical vignettes to explore further the issue of patients who end their treatment precipitately, often in an unplanned and abrupt way. Suddenly the analyst may find their patient wanting to reduce the number of sessions each week or wanting to finish their treatment with some degree of urgency.

The urgency usually has in it a blend of real external factors, but these are invested with a desperate quality. This situation can be very distressing to the analyst or therapist and leads to much soul searching: 'What have I not understood?' 'What have I done wrong?' If the patient wants to reduce the number of sessions each week, as in the case of Ms K, my second clinical example, the analyst is left wondering 'Is this the right thing to do or should I hold out for the more intensive treatment that gives much more oppor-tunity to understand what is happening, even if this risks the patient breaking off altogether?' The analyst is left wondering what to do when the patient wants to abruptly end their treatment ostensibly because of pressing external events, rather than the termination developing naturally out of the analysis. This was the situation for my third clinical example, Mr L. While it is entirely right that a patient should, and of course may, end their treatment whenever they wish, it remains our task to try and understand the state of mind involved in that event.

Clinical illustrations

Ms J

Ms J was in her late 30s and had ended her relationship with an older, authoritarian and controlling man. She had an elder brother who had died when she was a few months old. After working through a great deal of pain about this in her treatment she became somewhat freer of the burden of trying to be a replacement child. She seemed to develop a more lively and engaged involvement with her treatment and in the developments in her external life. With a lot of effort, she applied for a promotion in her work that would give her a substantial opportunity for professional development. This brought her into a closer relationship with me in her professional capacity and although anxious about this she seemed to feel more depen-dent and involved in her treatment. In the session after hearing that she had been finally offered the promotion she told me that she had heard someone calling her in the street. She realised it was the man with whom she had ended the relationship. She crossed the road to speak to him and their relationship resumed despite her many crippling doubts and uncertainties. She felt unable to resist his charms and demands, especially when he became very ill and seemed to need her even more than ever. On his insistence, because of his illness, Ms J gave up her promotion. Increasingly in her treatment, I found myself left with her doubts and uncertainty about the usefulness of our analytic task as she became more and more convinced that she had no choice but to continue the relationship with her older, ill partner, which, by definition, seemed to her to mean dispensing with many other opportunities.

Around this time she reported a dream:

> She looked over the top of a cliff and she could see a couple lying dead at the bottom of a cliff and Ms J walked away from the scene.

From her associations it became clear that this couple represented Ms J and me and our work together, which seemed to have become deadened and useless and which she was now walking away from. Also she was walking away from her promotion at work, which she now thought about disdainfully and as 'not for her', despite having worked so hard for it. The couple at the bottom of the cliff seemed a dead and therefore unavailable parental couple who had fallen over the cliff, she and I in our therapeutic endeavour who could not stop the patient – her – from walking away. Some weeks after this dream, Ms J ended her analysis to care for her increasingly ill partner. Due to her age, Ms J and I both knew that she was sacrificing her wish to have a baby but she felt this was just the way it had to be. In her last session with me she told me, for the first time, that she always slept with a photograph of her long-dead brother on her bedside table. I was surprised and shocked to learn of this at such a late point in her treatment. I thought Ms J was giving me, as she left her treatment, a photograph of herself as my dead patient, who had not been able to grow up and flourish with my analytic care. She was showing me how she could not leave her brother in her mind to die, despite all our work in this area, but had to struggle continuously, and vainly, for his resurrection. The pain and despair about this was left residing in me.

For Ms J, her partner and her long-dead brother represented her own projected and split-off needs and demands, which she actually hated but felt utterly bound to. The more she hated them, the more these damaged and destroyed external figures, also representing internal figures, controlled and dominated her. Ms J had hated her mother's attachment to and idealisation of her dead brother as she felt that she could never match up to the perfections of this 'golden' and, as she felt, preferred child. Her hatred of her dead brother seemed to paradoxically tie her into identifying with him as an object who did not grow or develop. As part of her identification with the 'golden' child was the unconscious need to bring to life the dead brother, now represented by the ill partner. Her guilt for the damage she unconsciously felt she had done to her internal and external objects with her hatred of them seemed too much for her to face as well as her despair that she could not repair her damaged objects to a sufficiently high standard. It was as if a delicate balance between her life and death instincts became unsettled at the moment that life was there to be painfully lived, represented by the new job. Living life would mean for Ms J facing her guilt about moving on herself, leaving her old, ill and needy partner and relinquishing, internally, her vain attempts to resurrect her dead brother.

To grow and develop in her analysis meant Ms J facing her vulnerability, that she was the needy one and dependent on her analyst to support and sustain her in her new development. When in her treatment Ms J was facing the potential for healthier object relations this seemed to provoke a vicious attack such that our therapeutic and potentially creative coupling was to be left, as in her dream, to die at the bottom of the cliff while she walked away. As if, an Iago-like aspect of herself had triumphed over the potential creative coupling of Othello and Desdemona.

Ms K

Ms K was a fragile and needy young woman who was under tremendous external and internal pressure to reduce the frequency of her sessions. I felt reluctant to agree that this was the best thing for her. At the time of the following dream she had decided that she was going to bring her treatment to an end. Ms K laughed as she told me her dream:

> She was in an American supermarket where a robbery was taking place, innocent hostages were being taken and eventually she too was taken hostage. Somebody told her that the gangsters break limbs, they really were dangerous and she could get killed. She thought that this wasn't serious. She was taken into a room with the other hostages but she still doubted the seriousness of the hostage takers. The room was like a staff common room which she said had features a bit like the analytic consulting room. She thought about lifting a blind to see if she could contact people in the outside world or escape but it was too dangerous because if the hostage takers saw her they might kill her.

The patient's associations to the dream were that the gangster, hostage takers in the American supermarket were like film characters and as such she found them funny. As she told me the dream I was impressed with its filmic quality and also her laughing dismissal of the dream. I thought that she was running in her mind a film version of her analysis that she did not take seriously but very much wanted me to believe. It also gave her an excited gratification as she laughed about it: the dream was not to be taken seriously as a dream to be analysed but presented with an air of mocking anyone who, like a psychoanalyst, might take her dream seriously. I thought there was a version that she did want me to take seriously, which was that the consulting room was a cruel place where hostages were taken and limbs were broken and from where she could not escape. This seemed to me to be an Iago-like idea, mischievous and corrosive, whose purpose was to undermine both me as her analyst and the analysis as a helpful place where she could gain understanding and grow emotionally. She knew that I thought she was not in a good state to be leaving her treatment and I knew that she felt this to be an imprisoning idea. It seemed to me that she was likening her psychoanalyst to the cruel hostage takers, as if I was holding her in the consulting room so that she was too frightened to lift the blind or leave. In her mind, my concern for her had become corrupted and altered into something cruel. I knew she had every intention of leaving her analysis shortly and despite telling me her dream a part of her was not at all interested in discussing it with me. She sowed seeds of doubt in my mind about the veracity of her analysis in order to undermine me and locate in me, rather than in herself, the cruel gangster that was destroying her treatment. She made herself out to be an innocent victim, a mere bystander to something violent and cruel. I interpreted to her that she was running in her mind a version of her analysis as a cruel place that she had to escape from but added that I was not sure how much she really believed this.

Ms K did not answer this and withdrew into her characteristic silence but then after a while she told me that she had remembered an earlier part of the dream, which was the reason she had gone to the supermarket in the first place:

> She was with her mother. Her mother said that she had been given £500 which she, the mother, could use as credit. Ms K was convinced that her mother was not entitled to this money but her mother insisted that she was and that she would pay it back sometime later. Despite her disapproval of her mother, Ms K had nevertheless gone into the supermarket to spend the money.

Ms K had no associations to this part of the dream. I thought her analyst was represented in the dream as a mother who had some wealth, £500, that she could borrow and pay back, but whom Ms K despised. Ms K had often told me of her hatred of being sent, as a little girl, by her mother to the local shop to 'buy things on tick'. She found it embarrassing and humiliating to have an irresponsible mother who had no money. In her analysis, Ms K had begun to experience me as an emotionally richer mother, different to her recollection of her mother and this had put her more in touch with her own emotional appetite; in the dream she had gone into the supermarket with the intention of using her mother's borrowed money. It seemed to me that it was just this appetite to use her mother's credit or her analyst's help that set in train a violent and murderous hostage-taking in her internal world, a wish to obliterate her perception of her own needs and the analyst who might help her think about, and therefore bear, these needs. Perhaps, too, Ms K found it difficult to give her analyst any credit for helping her, thereby enabling her to use this credit in the ordinary activity of shopping and feeding that enables life and development. The lure of a powerful feeling of superiority that is both all knowing and mocking is clear in the first part of Ms K's dream. I think it seemed more bearable for Ms K to sow mischief like Iago rather than suffer the pain and torment –powerful feelings of jealous rage followed immediately by overwhelming guilt – that drove Othello to kill Desdemona.

Mr L

Mr L reported the following dream at a time when he wanted to stop coming to his analysis or, at least, reduce the number of sessions he came to each week because he was convinced they were incompatible with his new job:

> He and a woman were sheltering in the house of a father-like figure. This father-like figure was keen to shelter them in a room along with his own family. It was very squashed in the room with all these people. The father figure was Italian and mafia-like. The patient said that in the dream he knew somebody was going to attack them all by puncturing the building they were in with bullets and he could not understand why this mafia-like, father figure was putting them all at risk by keeping them in the room. My patient then left the building himself.
>
> The dream had a second part in which the patient was in a comfortable place with his father. The father was very pleased that the patient was not rushing around any more. There was a wonderful feeling of togetherness and harmony.

Mr L's association to the dream was that he had not spoken to his father for sometime and his father was unaware that he had recently been promoted at work. The patient was frightened of receiving a telephone call to say that his father had had a heart attack. He did not think that his father would be at all pleased to hear of his new job as it meant he would not return to live near his parents.

In the first part of the dream the father is a grandiose figure who is claiming to be protective but is not. This father, like the patient's view of his analyst, offers well-meaning but ineffective shelter. In fact the building is punctured with bullets, just like the analysis, which was peppered with missed sessions, short sessions as he frequently arrived late and the prospect of a curtailment because he threatened to leave his analysis. There is reference, too, in the dream to the patient's hatred of the analyst's other patients and the analyst's family who he believes fill the consulting room making the patient feel squashed out and unattended to. The patient 'knows' of his own destructiveness towards the analysis and the way in which he punctures my attempts to provide analytic shelter for him. He simultaneously maintains the illusion that he is at risk when he has to share the consulting room with anyone else. For him it is the mafia-like father figure, his analyst, who puts them at risk by squashing everyone into the room and keeping them in the building. The patient has to leave, just as in reality he wanted to leave his analysis. But actually he leaves as in the second dream to something quite sterile, a deadly harmoniousness with his father where all activity has stopped and developments have been obliterated. My patient believes the news of his promotion will kill his actual father. In the dream I think something quite deadly is chosen in preference to risking staying in the building with a father who is trying to be protective of all his children, despite the constant attack of missed sessions and being late. Like Ms K, Mr L wanted to destroy his analysis and his analyst because to stay and face the precariousness of development seemed too risky. There is also a mischievous and undermining element in the dream, as in Ms K's dream described previously: the idea that the father figure is mafia-like nudges me into wondering if it is me who is really mafia-like, just treating my patient for my own ends and gain, for my own greedy grandiosity. So I, as Mr L's analyst, am left full of doubt about the veracity of my analytic intentions.

In the penultimate session of Mr L's analysis (although I did not know at the time that he would only come for one more session), he arrived late and very angry. Mr L started the session by telling me that he had gone to a cash dispenser and his card had been swallowed by the machine. He was furious as he said he was not overdrawn and if he hadn't been paid it was his employer's fault. He complained of the capitalist takeover with machines and computers everywhere. He was particularly indignant that he would need to use a cheque book to pay for a training course he was planning to attend. He then reported a dream:

> He found his lost credit card, but it was a new and shiny card, not his familiar well-used one.

I interpreted to Mr L, who had been late and missed half his session, that he had become the computerised machine that swallowed up the value that he gained from his analysis and that this left him feeling very disturbed and angry. He ignored what I said and told me that he had to stop coming to his analysis as it was too expensive. At that moment to engage with me really did feel too expensive to him as he only wanted to be given a new and shiny analysis rather than the familiar well used analysis that I offered him. The familiar analysis was in many ways more like a cheque book where transactions are visible, written out and with human contact and therefore subject to imperfections. Mr L, in this state of mind, despised what I had to offer and felt outraged. In his dream, he wanted a nice new shiny credit card analysis, not one that was used by him and other patients but one that produced riches, both material and emotional, out of the wall, on demand and accessible 24 hours a day, with no cost or human involvement. This is similar to his earlier dream when he did not want to be in an analysis with an analyst who had a room full of other patients, an analysis that he constantly punctured by his attacking bullets because it was too emotionally costly for him to face. The new shiny credit card, he felt, would give him the state of mind that he desired: powerful and invincible, not subject to the vicissitudes of human experience; feelings of hurt, rejection, jealousy, humiliation, smallness and doubt, as in his old, familiar, well-worn analysis. Mr L preferred, as Rosenfeld describes, to be in state of superiority and self-admiration at the cost of real life and development. Yet, this new shiny credit card state was very precarious as it could be swallowed arbitrarily by a terrifying, gobbling-up machine, the cash dispenser. Mr L experienced this machine as behaving randomly: it swallowed his credit card, representing any new developments in his analysis and it prevented him both from gaining any credit, in terms of internal resources, from his analysis, and also from giving me any credit for the work that we had done together in his analysis. I think the machine was the lure of a psychotic, dreamlike, deathly, timeless state where all capacity for thought and development had been obliterated and it was similar to the second part of his earlier dream when he was in harmony with his father, not rushing about anymore and not engaging in life by for example, finding a new job. At that moment, he experienced the gobbling-up cash dispenser as being located in the analyst and his analysis so he felt it was imperative to escape from the analysis before it swallowed him up.

I think that all the patients I have discussed found it difficult to give their analyst any credit for what had been, and what could yet be, achieved in treatment. In the analytic experiences that I have described, the analyst or therapist has to bear being left with feeling real doubt and uncertainty about themselves and psychoanalytic psychotherapy as a treatment: in effect the analyst is required to bear being annihilated. Like Desdemona's father any 'delight' we may have in our patient's growth and development is 'poisoned'. Just as we are deprived of any ordinary satisfaction with our work, so are these patients deprived of a fertile treatment. As Rosenfeld suggests, destructive narcissism is a form of undiffused death instinct, provoked by the release of life forces in the patient during treatment as represented, in the cases that I have outlined, by promotion, a new job and the sense that there is a richer emotional life to be experienced. Giving credit to the analysis and the patient's own life forces, as represented in their dependent involvement with their treatment, challenges their psychic equilibrium and provokes a deadly 'sneer'. As Iago executes the most terrible cruel revenge on Othello by sowing seeds of doubt about Desdemona's loyalty and love for him so our patients can mischievously sow seeds of doubt and uncertainty in their psychotherapist. This can be seen in the hostage taking in Ms K's dream and the ineffectual mafia father figure of Mr L's dream who makes false claims. The aim of this mischief is to wreck the potential, but fragile, creativity of the therapy, turning it from a viable endeavour into a dead couple at the bottom of the cliff as evidenced in Ms J's dream, deadly harmony with his father in

Mr L's dream or, as he reports in his penultimate session, a machine that swallows up credit and development.

The treatment therefore ends much as in the final exchange between Othello and Iago: Othello, dying, asks of Iago: 'Why he hath thus ensnar'd my soul and body?' Iago, chillingly impregnable, replies:

> Demand me nothing: what you know, you know:
> From this time forth I will never speak word.

References

Bion, W.R. (1967) *Second Thoughts: Selected Papers on Psychoanalysis*, London: Karnac

Freud, S. (1923) 'The ego and the id', *Standard Edition 19*, London: Hogarth Press
—— (1937) 'Analysis terminable and interminable', *Standard Edition 23*, London: Hogarth Press

O'Shaughnessy, E. (1981) 'A clinical study of a defensive organisation', *International Journal of Psychoanalysis* 62: 359–69

Rosenfeld, H. (1986) 'Destructive narcissism and the death instinct' in *Impasse and Interpretation*, London: Tavistock Publications

Segal, H. (1993) 'On the clinical usefulness of the death instinct', *International Journal of Psychoanalysis* 74: 55–61

Spillius, E. Bott (ed.) (1988) *Melanie Klein Today: Developments in Theory and Practice, Volume 1*, London: Routledge

Steiner, J. (1993) *Psychic Retreats*, London: Routledge

Chapter 14

Absence and absent-mindedness

Mary Thomas

Introduction

In this chapter, I will explore some of the difficulties of working with absent patients, that is, patients who absent themselves physically or psychologically from the consulting room while being 'in' psychotherapy or psychoanalysis. A difficulty in engaging in the therapeutic work may be expressed through frequent lateness and absence from sessions. For many patients who are 'difficult to reach' (Joseph 1975), the analytic container is experienced more as an abusive, entrapping claustrum, from which absence is necessary for survival, rather than a place for development. Absence may function to defend and protect the patient from exposure in the too-bright glare of the analytic work, but absence can also constitute an aggressive attack on the analytic container and the mind and function of the psychotherapist.

I explore some of my thinking about absence as a defence against, and as a partial solution to, the anxieties aroused in the therapeutic relationship and also the importance for the psychotherapist of processing his or her counter-transference responses in order to develop an understanding of the meaning of the patient's absences. Survival of the deadliness and despair that absent patients may evoke in their therapist is regarded as a key factor in the work. Emanuel states the importance of the survival of the therapist in the face of the meaninglessness that can be engendered by unreachable patients:

> Whilst we all have experience of trying to reach unreachable patients, survival of the mind and interest of the therapist in these circumstances seems a key issue in working with these phenomena . . . what is being transferred is a strong sense of non-being, of ceasing to exist in the room, of trying to find something to hold on to, whether it be psycho-analytic theory, one's supervisor, analyst, whatever. Survival itself seems to be what requires to be understood.
>
> (Emanuel 2001: 1080)

The effect of the patient's absence on the therapist

For the purposes of this chapter, I shall focus on one patient, a professional woman in her mid-30s in three times weekly psychotherapy and shall refer to her as the 'absent patient'. However, I am aware of the paradoxical nature of this title as, on balance, she was probably more physically present than absent and, in some senses was more present in her absence than in her presence, in the sense that she absented herself psychically and emotionally when physically present. Some patients in psychoanalysis or psychotherapy may occasionally be absent, or have periods of absence, but are otherwise actively engaged in a joint analytic endeavour. For these patients, periods of absence, because they are remarkable, can become objects of curiosity and exploration. When Ogden advocates that his supervisees explore their responses to an absent patient, I think he has in mind a less persistent or virulent form of absence from analysis, that is, one that can be engaged with more readily:

> I operate under the assumption that the patient's physical absence creates a specific form of psychological effect in the analyst and in the analysis, and that the analytic process continues despite the analysand's physical absence. In this way, the specific meanings of the patient's *presence in his absence* are transformed into analytic objects to be fully experienced, lived with, symbolised, understood and made part of the analytic discourse.
>
> (Ogden 1999: 137, emphasis added)

Ogden describes how he asks supervisees to write process notes for all sessions including those that the patient fails to attend. When supervising he wants to hear about all of the analyst's moment-to-moment thoughts, feelings and sensations and reveries during the patient's absences.

In contrast, those patients who are persistently or relentlessly absent present different technical and emotional problems for the psychoanalyst or psychotherapist. One is left struggling with questions such as, 'What is being communicated in this particular absence?' 'Is this particular absence due to a failure of attunement?' 'Is it a response to a clumsy interpretation or an interpretation that came too close to the patient's core pain or an interpretation that was too late/too early/way off the mark?' But when the absences begin to accumulate, unmitigated by sufficient presence of the patient to jointly explore the potential meaning of the absences, then the analyst is left holding the belief and doubt in the analytic process and one's curiosity and faith in the process can begin to erode.

When my 'absent patient' expressed frustration and impotence about her own lateness and persistent absence, the communication seemed to be something like this: 'I cannot control this (it's in control of me), so just accept it and *don't make anything of it* because to point it out will point out my failings and I am already beating myself up for being a failure.' Riesenberg-Malcolm (1999) suggests that patients who use self-punishment as a defence against a painful awareness of the damaged state of their internal objects, may operate on the principle that 'no change' will provide them with safety from pain and disintegration.

The accumulation of my patient's absences led to a sense of their embodying a monolithic impenetrability in which it was difficult to gain a handhold or a foothold. This monolith could be understood as a petrified version of a resistance to analysis and development and was reflected in my patient likening her difficulties in getting to the third session of the week (the session from which she was most often absent and the session in which she located her potential for change) to trying to push a huge boulder up a steep hill. The boulder kept getting bigger and bigger, the hill steeper and steeper. There was often a sense in the work that the boulder might roll back down the hill and flatten us both and that the analytic work and relationship could be destroyed at any minute.

In the work with the 'absent patient', the experience of waiting, not knowing whether the patient was going to come or not and the accumulation of absences came to feel like a kind of torture. It became more difficult to hold onto analytic thinking in the face of the 'nothingness' of the patient's absence. While waiting for the patient I felt like a character in a Samuel Beckett play, *Waiting for Godot*, trying to hang onto a reason for carrying on, for holding the 'going on being' of the analytic process.

I found myself becoming especially interested in Beckett's work when thinking about the 'absent patient'. His attempts to find some humanity, humour and reason to go on in the face of apparent meaninglessness and despair offers some parallels to the psychotherapist struggling with the necessity of 'going on being' in the face of the patient's destructive attacks on contact and linking. In *Waiting for Godot*, it is the *waiting* that provides the structure and purpose for the two main characters to go on living. But waiting for what? For rescue? For relief from responsibility? For meaning? David Mayers, in his fascinating study of similarities in the work of Beckett and Bion (Beckett was in analysis with Bion for two years in the 1930s), refers to Billie Whitelaw's autobiography where she describes how Beckett encouraged her to 'play' a state of mind, rather than a character. He points out the parallel in Bion's advice that we think of ourselves, in the consulting room, as confronting not a character but a state of mind (Mayers 2000: 194). I came to think of my increasingly despairing *state of mind* in the face of the patient's persistent absence as the projectively identified *state of mind* of the absent patient, and that there was a despairing baby self that the patient needed to absent herself from.

The container and the claustrum

So far I have considered some aspects of the underlying causes of the patient's absences in terms of resistance to change and development and repudiation of the needy infantile self, but these can only be partial explanations and do not convey adequately the patient's immense psychic suffering, albeit blanked off, which led her into psychotherapy. In psychotherapy, I believe she was unconsciously seeking a container in which she would be enabled to find her own mind. However, as the transference developed she experienced me as the narcissistic and domineering mother of her infancy leading her to experience the potential space of the therapeutic container as an entrapping claustrum that threatened her existence. Absence from the therapy felt crucial for *her* survival.

Roger Willoughby (2001) in his paper on the claustrum as pathological container, outlines the development of the psychoanalytic concepts of the container and the claustrum. In Bion's model of the 'container-contained' the infant's bad feelings (or beta elements) are projected into the good breast container, processed and detoxified there by the receptive mother's reverie (love and understanding) or alpha function and reintrojected in their modified form (or alpha element). If all goes well, the infant is helped to develop its own capacity for thinking and toleration of feelings, and meaning is created. This symbolic and generative notion of the container-contained is contrasted by the 'anti-developmental concrete retreat that is the claustrum' (Willoughby 2001: 917). The claustrum is a place (or state of mind) that is against meaning and against development that is 'making nothing out of something', as contrasted with the container, 'making something out of nothing'.

Willoughby describes how the term 'claustrum' originally meant a boundaried space and 'cloister', the enclosed living space of a monastery is a derivation from it. Cloister was used as a synonym for the womb and the term 'cloister' together with 'phobia' formed the roots of the term 'claustrophobia' (fear of the womb). The psychoanalytic usage and understanding of claustrophobia and the claustrum has varied in the Freudian, Kleinian, and Independent groups. Freud observed the 'remarkable dread that many people have of being buried alive' (quoted by Willoughby 2001: 918) and believed that the actual birth experience, and being separated from the mother, was the first experience of anxiety and formed the basis for all phobias, including claustrophobia. Ferenczi regarded claustrophobia as a defence against the wish to return to the womb, whereas Klein saw it more as a fear of being shut up inside mother's dangerous body. Klein refined her understanding of claustrophobia as: 'projective identification into the mother leading to an anxiety of imprisonment inside her; and reintrojection resulting in a feeling that inside oneself one is hemmed in by resentful internal objects' (quoted in Willoughby 2001: 920) She also wrote that:

[P]rojective identification may result in the fear that the lost part of the self will never be recovered because it is buried in the object . . . besides the fear of being imprisoned inside the mother, I have found that another contributory factor to claustrophobia is the fear relating to the inside of one's own body and the dangers threatening there. To quote Milton's lines, 'Thou art become (O worst imprisonment) the dungeon of thyself'.

(quoted by Willoughby 2001: 920)

Meltzer was particularly interested in the geography of object relationships and elaborated his notion of compartmentalised dwelling places for parts of the infantile self. He described the claustrum as 'a refuge for infantile parts of the personality from mental pain and individuation' (Willoughby 2001: 925), and entry into it was by intrusive projective identification. It was a pathological organisation that was similar to Steiner's 'psychic retreats' (1993) and Rosenfeld's 'mafia gang' (1987) of destructive narcissism. Meltzer defined three different types of claustrum, the mother's head-breast, genitals and rectum and dwelling in a particular 'compartment' signified specific pathologies. When intrusively entered by the infantile self, these 'compartments', although attractive from the outside, inevitably become prisons. While offering some narcissistic gratifications and freedom from pain, relationship and development, the price for claustral dwellers is a mindless existence in a sado-masochistic and cynical state, with the constant fear of evacuation into a delusional 'no-where'.

I think the absent patient's internal conflict about her therapy, which led her to absent herself as her only means of psychic survival, ran something like this: she was unconsciously searching for a benign therapeutic container, akin to a cloister, where there would be potential for quiet reflection and protection from the immediate demands of the external world. This container would also have the quality of a transitional space (Winnicott 1971) where there is potential for play and creative linking of ideas. Instead, she experienced the therapeutic container as a claustrum, where she experienced herself as being buried alive, entombed in a maternal necropolis (Green 1986), trapped in mother's dangerous body and with the constant fear of being violently expelled, as in a traumatic birth experience, into a frightening nothingness. Her fear, constantly reiterated, was that the therapy would deprive her of her hiding places, which would mean no escape from entombment with the (dead) mother. The meaninglessness of existence in the claustrum, and in the maternal necropolis, was conveyed in the patient's use of language, which was repetitive and empty. There was often nothing on her mind, her mind was blank or she could not think of anything to say. This position is captured by Julia Kristeva when she links depression to the loss of language and of being buried alive:

The speech of the depressed is to them like an alien skin; melancholy persons are foreigners in their maternal tongue. They have lost the meaning – the value – of their mother tongue for want of losing the mother. The dead language they speak, which foreshadows their suicide, conceals a Thing buried alive. The latter, however, will not be translated in order that it not be betrayed; it shall remain walled up within the crypt of inexpressible affect, anally harnessed, with no way out.

(1941: 53)

Sekoff, elaborating on André Green's concept of the dead mother syndrome, describes how the dead mother keeps the child/patient in thrall, in a half alive state, *entombed* in her embrace, and writes: 'Within her tight embrace the entombed child finds solace, a shelter that offers the certainties of death over the vagaries of life' (1999: 115). According to Green, the enlivenment and resuscitation of the bereft, depressed or absent mother becomes the life task (or prison sentence) of the subject, who remains entombed frozen and distanced from any life in the world. I believe that my patient, in the transference, experienced the therapy as a claustrum in which she was buried alive and from which she had to absent herself in order to survive. I wondered about the boulder she described, which she had to push up the hill on the way to the third session of the week and its resonance with the boulder at the opening of Christ's tomb. The boulder may not have been merely a concrete version of her resistance to the therapy but also a representation of her entombment with her internal mother, from which it was a huge effort to break free.

Absence as attack on the therapist's mind

There was a peculiarly tortuous quality as I waited session after session, not knowing if the patient was going to arrive or not. Waiting was particularly tortuous during the early morning sessions, which my patient often reported sleeping through, while I felt sleep deprived. I found myself experiencing alternating states of hope and despair, leading, at times when the patient was frequently absent, to more enduring states of despair and a questioning of the meaning and value of the analytic work. Betty Joseph (1982) writing about patients with an addiction to near-death, describes how some patients will try to create despair in the analyst and provoke him into becoming critical or verbally sadistic towards the patient. If they succeed in creating despair or in getting themselves hurt they may triumph at the analyst's loss of analytic balance and capacity to understand but the therapeutic work fails. I noticed that while I waited I developed little rituals like preparing hot drinks or snacks, perhaps to soothe and compensate myself for the attacks on my analytic function or perhaps to retaliate through oral aggression and then sometimes felt some resentment if the patient arrived and interrupted my compensatory ritual.

Fakhry Davids (2002) describes his attempts to dedicate himself to thinking about his absent patient for the duration of the missed sessions but wondered if this was partly a denial of the absence of the patient and also found that his unconscious was not so cooperative that his thoughts and feelings about the patient would occur within the 50-minutes session time:

> Why is the patient's absence so difficult to bear? I think it is because, in order to work well, we must have some narcissistic investment in our work. Patients sense this commitment from our palpable satisfaction, often subtly conveyed, when things go well. This is different from a transference for it presents an aspect of our real selves, which patients can put to use for their own purposes, knowing that they can touch us by doing so.
>
> (Davids 2002: 33)

Davids describes his counter-transference responses to a patient who was persistently late or absent, how these changed over time and the understanding he achieved about the meaning of the patient's absence. He found that, while waiting for his patient he could only do mindless administrative work, not truly creative work like writing a paper. He came to understand his own guilt about how he 'wasted time' on routine, on mindless things, as a reflection of his patient's unconscious and unbearable guilt about his wasted years picking (internal) fights with his parents and the damage done to his internal objects. Davids acknowledges the narcissistic blow to the analyst of a patient's persistent absence and the attack on the analyst's investment in, and commitment to, the analytic work that the absence involves. He advocates the necessity of the analyst acknowledging their own vulnerability and of surviving the narcissistic blow in order to engage in the much more complex task of paying attention to their counter-transference responses and observing them over time in order to try to reach some understanding of the unconscious meaning of the patient's absence. What Davids implicitly conveys but does not elaborate is the attack on the analyst's creativity, which inhibits him from doing any creative work or thinking while waiting for the patient. This parallels the patient's attack on his/her own creativity and on the potential for creative intercourse between analyst and patient.

When my patient was present it was an agonising struggle for her to speak. She felt there was nothing to say and often reported that her mind was blank. Despite leading a busy and relatively successful professional life, she told me very little of her daily existence. I was starved of anecdote and detail and was left full of fantasies about her internal and external worlds. I had to tolerate the frustration of not being allowed to know her, of being kept out and of little creative intercourse being allowed to happen between us.

Sabbadini (1991) explores the meaning of silence in analysis, how it can be overloaded with meaning as resistance when specific instances of silence with specific patients can have very many and complex meanings, including silence as a container for words, words that cannot be spoken. Similarly absence may be thought of primarily as a resistance to analytic work, but its meaning in relation to a specific patient cannot be reduced simply to this and needs to be understood through exploration of both analyst's and supervisor's counter-transference responses. Silence may be thought of as a kind of absence and absence as a kind of silence, but the patient's silence during a session in which they are present is very different to the silence of the absent patient. The silent but present patient may be conveying some resistance to, or attack on, the analytic work but this may be countered by the unconscious hope or belief in the work that their physical presence embodies. The persistently absent patient gives the therapist less to go on and the value of the analytic work can be more difficult to hold onto. The psychotherapist is thrown back more on her own resources, both internal and external. Supervision can be crucial to enable the therapist to engage in a dialogue to explore her counter-transference responses and to try to reflect on the meaning of the patient's absence, when absence can present one with powerful feelings of meaninglessness. It is this sense of meaninglessness that can be felt as an attack on one's analytic mind and function (making nothing out of something), when one's creative and professional strivings are to make, or seek, meaning (making something out of nothing).

The accumulation of absences had an eroding effect on my belief in the analytic work and left me feeling I was being cruelly tantalised. Explanations for her absences or lateness were rarely offered and any probing on my part about this led to a defensive self-berating by the patient, which seemed to put her further out of reach. Like the two main characters in *Waiting for Godot*, I needed to tolerate a huge amount of uncertainty and not knowing.

Absence as negative therapeutic reaction

The persistent absence of a patient could be thought of as a particular type of negative therapeutic reaction. Victor Sedlak describes Freud's Wolf Man as an example of the silent way in which the negative therapeutic reaction is often expressed and comments that a therapist who is able to tolerate overt expressions of aggression can be undone by a covert silent resistance:

> [I]n a letter to Ferenczi written after his first consultation with the Wolf Man, he noted with pleasure that this new patient was an interesting case who disclosed in the first hour that he thought Freud to be a 'Jewish swindler' and that he already entertained thoughts of 'shitting on his analyst's head' (Gay 1988: p. 287). This conscious verbalization of

his patient's aggression did not perturb Freud; what finally undid Freud's resolve to do as he advised others to do, that is, keep on analysing, was the constant repudiation of his work – one might say, the daily shitting on his head by the Wolf Man.

(Sedlak 1997: 30)

Sedlak suggests that Freud enacted something in response to this negative therapeutic reaction, rather than maintaining his analytic function, by terminating the Wolf Man's treatment prematurely. Ignes Sodre (2005) observed that some patients seem to specialise in almost invisible but serial negative therapeutic reactions that are aimed at maintaining the status quo, producing in the analysis an atmosphere of 'nothing-ever-happens-here' and an illusion of a-temporality. She advises the analyst to remember that there is no such thing as the abolition of time and that this 'nothing is a very particular kind of something'. My absent patient's absolute belief was that nothing would ever change in her life and this was reflected in what felt, at times, like a stubborn insistence that nothing was going to happen in her therapy.

Thinking of negative therapeutic reactions as attempts to *kill* time, *kill* change, *kill* the possibility of something creative happening between therapist and patient, points to their destructive and aggressive nature. When Freud (quoted by Rosenfeld 1987: 96) introduced the term he regarded it as related to the death instinct and its silent influence, a mute and hidden force that opposes all progress and that involves a deep preoccupation with death and destructiveness. Rosenfeld (1987) outlines how many psychoanalysts, observing chronic and often hidden resistances to the analytic work, followed Freud in developing an understanding of negative therapeutic reactions, identifying in the operation elements of envy, guilt, the superego, and narcissistic omnipotence. These analysts observed that patients often experienced help from the analyst or therapist, in the form of a good interpretation for example, as a narcissistic blow that exposed unwanted feelings of dependency and need. This sometimes led the patient to retaliate by belittling the therapist in a bid to assert their own superiority. Riviere (1936) thought the negative therapeutic reaction may be a response to an incorrect interpretation rather than a good one and she also cautioned against overdoing the analysis of aggressive impulses as she believed that nothing would more surely lead to a negative therapeutic reaction than an exclusive focus on the patient's aggression.

Rosenfeld (1987) noted from his own clinical practice and from his thinking on the nature of narcissistic object relating that it was not surprising that negative therapeutic reactions are most likely to occur after a session where the patient acknowledges feeling better and that the analysis is helping him. This was a noticeable feature of my work with 'the absent patient', where her absences predictably increased following a session where we made some good contact and she allowed more creative linking and insight to happen. This left me with a feeling that any progress or change had to be demolished, although my patient's sense of her increased absence was that it was beyond her control. It partly served to slow things down when things were going too quickly for her. If things progressed 'too quickly' in the therapy, she argued, the end of therapy would arrive before she was ready to leave. It was as if she could put off the inevitable end of the therapy and the loss she would experience, by imposing a series of lesser losses – the absences – which at least were more under her omnipotent control. There was also the element of a pre-emptive defence against loss; if she did not allow much good contact between us then she would have less to lose. My response to the absences, the 'constant shitting on my head' was an erosion of hope and belief in the analytic work.

Absence as defence of vulnerable self

In this section I want to return to and highlight the 'claustro-agoraphobic' dilemma (Rey in Steiner 1993: 53) that many patients in psychotherapy struggle with and that was a significant feature of the absent patient's psychopathology. This dilemma is manifest in rapid oscillation between claustrophobic and agoraphobic anxieties. According to Fairbairn (in Willoughby 2001), the infantile self oscillated between fears of engulfment (claustrophobia) or isolation (agoraphobia) and the 'claustrophobic self' fears it will be trapped with its primary object. This is akin to Glasser's (1979) notion of the core complex, where the subject moves constantly between the fantasy of merger with an idealised mother, the subsequent fear of being engulfed and annihilated and the narcissistic withdrawal into self-sufficiency that leads to feelings of abandonment and isolation. I have discussed my patient's experience of the therapy container as a terrifying claustrum that she believed she had to absent herself from for fear of being engulfed and wiped out and how this was at the cost of isolation and lack of change and development. For this patient, and others in psychotherapy, absenting themselves, whether physically or psychically, provides a temporary 'solution' to the claustro-agoraphobic dilemma. It seems to offer a no-place to be, although too prolonged a stay there can become claustrophobic in itself. These no-places are often experienced as hiding places and may have the characteristics of what Steiner (1993) observed as 'psychic retreats'.

Steiner (1993) defined a psychic retreat as providing the patient with an area of relative peace and protection from strain, akin to the idea of the cloister, when meaningful contact with the analyst was experienced as threatening. While transient withdrawals of this kind are understandable, evidence of more serious pathological organisations, or systems of defences, is conveyed by patients who turn to psychic retreats habitually and excessively. Steiner states that the analyst may identify psychic retreats as states of mind in which the patient is cut off, stuck and out of reach, whereas the patient's view of the retreat is revealed in the pictorial or dramatised image of how the retreat is experienced unconsciously, e.g. as a house, a cave or a fortress. It can also be represented as a business organisation, a totalitarian government or a mafia-like gang and the tyrannical and perverse elements in such descriptions may be idealised as well as feared (Steiner 1993: 2). While a psychic retreat may provide relief from anxiety and pain, it is at the cost of isolation and withdrawal. Some patients may be distressed by their reliance on their psychic retreats and others accept it with resignation, even defiance and triumph, 'so that it is the analyst who has to carry the despair associated with the failure to make contact' (Steiner 1993: 2).

The 'absent patient' showed a great dependence on her psychic retreats, whether the retreat was located in her physical absence or in a state of mind. Although her communications in the consulting room were characterised by states of blankness and psychic absence and a lack of mental representation – nothing going on, nothing changing – she occasionally spontaneously produced very vivid images of her mental states from her unconscious. One such image that came to my patient early in the therapy was of *mushrooms in the dark*: a dark hiding place where some sort of life could develop, sustained by rotting and decaying matter. This seemed to represent something important about the omnipotent and self-sufficient nature of her psychic retreat that was set apart from the therapy container. The element of decay appeared in another vivid image that came to her mind in the latter stages of her therapy and seemed to represent a slightly different psychic retreat. In this scenario, she is in the sea clinging to a rotting piece of wood after a shipwreck. She can see the shore, knowing she will survive if she just swims to the shore, but instead she clings to the rotting wood, knowing that she will drown. She seemed to be choosing the omnipotent certainty of death (no change) rather than risk the uncertainty and pain of living. Joyce McDougall described some patients who were affect-less and whose psychoanalytic process seemed to stagnate for long periods of time: 'The analysands themselves frequently complained that "nothing was happening" in their analytic adventure, yet each clung to his analysis like a drowning man to a life preserver' (1989: 91). McDougall first coined the term 'anti-analysands in analysis' to describe patients who fiercely opposed the analysis of anything to do with their inner psychic world. She later reviewed her thinking on this saying that, in her earlier paper, she inadequately explored the depth of despair and experience of inner death that lay behind the suffering and angry resistance to psychic change of this group of patients: 'They believe profoundly that change can only be for the worse. Immobility is felt to be the only protection against a return to an unbearable and inexpressible traumatic state' (1989: 93).

Despite the rather bleak nature of my patient's retreat, in which she preferred to cling to the rotting wood of omnipotent self-sufficiency even though she knew this would lead to certain death, the shoreline has appeared on the horizon as a hopeful sign of life and object relating. I thought of 'the shore' as her momentary recognition that the therapeutic relationship may offer a more hopeful alternative to the deadliness of her psychic retreat, even though she stubbornly refused to swim towards it at that point.

The terror that the potential of the psychotherapeutic relationship aroused in my patient was illustrated by a memory of her traumatic experience of visiting the dissecting room in a hospital mortuary. Initially, she found it impossible to think about the link I made between this trauma and her experience in my consulting room but tentatively came back to it over the following three years until she was able to speak of it more fully. At this point she told me that, on that visit to the mortuary, she had seen a severed head lying in a sink in the dissecting room. She was horrified by the lack of respect and cruelty that the severed head represented to her. This mortuary visit was like descending into hell. She contrasted the callousness conveyed to her by the severed head in the mortuary with the respect and care accorded to the patients in the hospital above. It was as if she had stumbled on a cruel and inhuman underworld, the shadow side of the benign, caring environment of the hospital. I believe she was also conveying her anxiety about the psychotherapy relationship. Was there a cruel and sadistic aspect to this apparently benign relationship? Would the cruel and sadistic side of her be exposed in the consulting room?

I came to think of the dissecting room in the mortuary as signifying the perverse container, the claustrum that the psychotherapy came to embody, at times, for my patient, and from which she had to absent herself repeatedly. I understood my tortured and despairing states of mind as a reflection (or projective identification) of my patient's cruel and tortured internal world. She was preoccupied by all the people she had ever known who had died and whether she had caused them to die through her neglect. As she spoke of all those she had neglected I think she was conveying her (unconscious) guilt about her treatment of me, the effect her absences were having on me and on the quality of our relationship.

Absence as communication

I believe the patient's unconscious aim was to find a transitional space in therapy where she could develop a mind of her own. But her predominant anxiety – that I, as the domineering mother in the transference, would bulldoze her and rob her of her hiding places – led her to believe that the potential transitional space offered in the therapeutic relationship was a dangerous claustrum where she would be buried alive. I heard her accounts of her mother's invasion of her private spaces and, by implication, her mind, as warning me against a too intense or direct contact which she equated with invasion and annihilation. But, paradoxically, in her description of her emotionally distant father, she also warned me of the danger of too little emotional contact with her. This patient's internal landscape gradually unfolded as being inhabited by rather polarised internal parental objects – the over-intrusive mother and the distant father. In her internal world, she was left with nowhere to go or be and nowhere to develop a sense of self with a mind of her own. Her horror at seeing the severed head in the mortuary stirred up a frightening recognition of herself as being psychically beheaded, as not having a mind, of being, quite literally, *absent minded*. Perhaps she also had the glimmering of a recognition of the violent severing inside herself between her thinking and feeling self (her 'body') and her public and compliant persona (her 'head'), as well as the links she severed in the therapeutic work.

Despite, or more likely *because of*, my continuing counter-transference of lingering in the claustrum dungeon of the dissecting room/torture chamber, my patient eventually began to report on noticing some change and progress in her life outside the consulting room. She told me how she was starting to stand up for herself with her friends and was not letting them take advantage of her as much as she had in the past. She also started to think about leaving the caring profession that she felt she had entered to alleviate her sense of herself as bad. She reported that she was overeating less and that food no longer provided her with an escape and relief: her bingeing was not functioning in the same way as a refuge or psychic retreat. These reports of progress outside of the consulting room seemed in stark contrast to the continuing experience of stalemate and agony inside the room. It was as if one of us had to be consigned to the darkness of the dungeon for the other one to progress and thrive and as if the development of one was at the expense of the other. I think this illustrates something of the deprivation she suffered in early infancy when she felt she was consigned to the dungeon so that the maternal object could thrive. This dynamic, where one thrived at the expense of the other, seemed to be present in my writing about my work with this patient. Around this time my patient told me about the bitterness and resentment she felt towards a female colleague, with whom she had worked on a joint piece of research. The original aim had been that they would write up the research together. However, it was her colleague who wrote up the research and presented it at a conference attended by my patient. She felt that the colleague was developing her career at my patient's expense, robbing her of her creativity. The parallel with my publishing the 'joint research' of the therapy with the absent patient is obvious. In the process of writing up the work with this patient, I was initially gripped by 'publication anxiety' (Britton 1997: 14) where publication evokes oedipal anxieties with associated feelings of betrayal, guilt and shame and also fear of retaliation by a third party for advertising possession of knowledge. The ethical dilemmas of approaching the (by now former) patient for permission to publish seemed unthinkable and insurmountable. It would be too damaging to the patient, too much of a betrayal. This brought on a paralysis of mind and thinking (and writing) that seemed to parallel the patient's prohibition on creativity and her internal conflicts in the psychotherapy, where exposure, or 'publication' of her self was experienced as potentially too damaging, but hiding in the psychic retreats of her absent states led to paralysis and lack of development.

I do not think that my patient reached a point of experiencing the therapeutic relationship as mutually gratifying and collaborative or a 'joint piece of research'. However, I think there were signs of more capacity for object relating in her move from the self-sufficient psychic retreat of the *mushrooms in the dark*, to the *sink with the rotting wood or swim to shore* retreat, in that an alternative way of life and relating was appearing in her unconscious, albeit on a distant horizon. The dead tree that is the only feature in an otherwise bleak landscape in *Waiting for Godot*, echoing the rotting wood in my patient's sink-or-swim psychic retreat, sprouts four or five leaves towards the end of the play. These slight signs of hope and growth are crucial in sustaining both patient and therapist in the analytic endeavour.

My patient's complaint that *I might as well have not been there*, which I understood as a complaint about her mother's narcissistic use of her that left her feeling she did not exist, was enacted in her therapy, concretely by her absences and lateness, and symbolically in her thwarting of contact or creative intercourse between us. Her refusal to be mother's perfect daughter was enacted in the transference as her unconscious refusal to be a good, cooperative or gratifying psychotherapy patient. Apart from the destructiveness inherent in this patient's refusal to allow much contact or creative intercourse between us, there is also a sense of it being a bid for life, the beginning of an attempt to establish a sense of identity and self. The aggression inherent in her refusal – I refuse, therefore I am – could be understood as a belated attempt to establish the 'me' from the 'not me' that was missing from her early development (Winnicott 1971: 93).

Conclusion

In this chapter, I have described the painstaking and difficult work of surviving the counter-transference with an inaccessible and persistently absent patient, where it seems that survival – of the deadliness and despair evoked by the absence and attack on the analytic work – by maintaining one's ability to think and hold the value of the analytic work is the most important and therapeutically useful function.

At the point at which this patient left her therapy there were signs that she was slowly emerging from her psychic retreats and risking more contact with me before retreating back to the safety of her hiding places. Her abrupt exit from the therapy felt like another violent severance of connection, reminiscent of the severed head in the dissecting room of the mortuary. It was as if her connection with me had to be violently severed by her leaving in order to convey to me something of her experience of the traumatising severance inside herself, an aspect of her internal conflict that could not yet be mentalised. Her state of mind and internal conflict was captured in Estragon's plea to Vladimir in Beckett's *Waiting for Godot* and perhaps conveys something of the paralysing conflict of the absent or 'unreachable' patient:

> *Estragon*: Don't touch me! Don't question me! Don't speak to me! Stay with me!

Postscript

The process of contacting the former patient to seek permission to publish has led to a more collaborative, post-psychotherapy phase of engagement that has enabled some reparative work to go on and has opened up the possibility of future analytic work.

References

Beckett, S. (1956) *Waiting for Godot*, London: Faber & Faber
Britton, R. (1997) 'Making the private public' in *The Presentation of Case Material in Clinical Discourse*, London: The Freud Museum
Davids, F.M. (2002) 'Surviving the empty couch' in *Between Sessions and Beyond the Couch*, J. Raphael-Leff (ed.), Colchester: University of Essex Press
Emanuel, R. (2001) 'A-void – an exploration of defences against sensing nothingness', *International Journal of Psychoanalysis* 82(6): 1069–84
Glasser, M. (1979) 'Some aspects of the role of aggression in the perversions' in *Sexual Deviation*, I. Rosen (ed.), Oxford: Oxford University Press
Green, A. (1986) 'The dead mother' in *On Private Madness*, London: Karnac
Joseph, B. (1975) 'The patient who is difficult to reach' in *Melanie Klein Today, Volume 2, Mainly Practice*, E. Bott Spillius (ed.), London: Routledge
—— (1982) 'Addiction to near-death' in *Melanie Klein Today, Volume 1, Mainly Theory*, E. Bott Spillius (ed.), London: Routledge
Kristeva, J. (1941) *Black Sun*, New York: Columbia Press
McDougall, J. (1989) *Theatres of the Body*, London: Free Association Books
Mayers, D. (2000) 'Bion and Beckett together', *British Journal of Psychotherapy* 17(2): 192–202
Ogden, T. (1999) 'Analysing forms of aliveness and deadness of the transference–

countertransference' in *The Dead Mother*, G. Kohon (ed.), London: Brunner-Routledge

Riesenberg-Malcolm, R. (1999) *On Bearing Unbearable States of Mind*, London: Routledge

Riviere, J. (1936) 'A contribution to the analysis of the negative therapeutic reaction', *International Journal of Psychoanalysis* 17: 304–20

Rosenfeld, H. (1987) *Impasse and Interpretation*, London: Routledge

Sabbadini, A. (1991) 'Listening to silence', *British Journal of Psychotherapy* 21(2): 229–40

Sedlak, V. (1997) 'Psychoanalytic supervision of untrained therapists' in *Supervision and Its Vicissitudes*, B. Martindale (ed.), London: Karnac

Sekoff, J. (1999) 'The undead: necromancy and the inner world' in *The Dead Mother*, G. Kohon (ed.), London: Brunner-Routledge

Sodre, I. (2005) '"As I was walking down the stair, I saw a concept which wasn't there . . ." Or, *après-coup*: A missing concept?', *International Journal of Psychoanalysis* 86(1): 7–10

Steiner, J. (1993) *Psychic Retreats*, London: Routledge

Willoughby, R. (2001) '"The dungeon of thyself": the claustrum as pathological container', *International Journal of Psychoanalysis* 82(5): 917–31

Winnicott, D. (1971) 'Mirror-role of mother and family in child development' in *Playing and Reality*, London: Tavistock Publications

Index